Working with

Children's Voice Disorders

Working with

Children's Voice Disorders

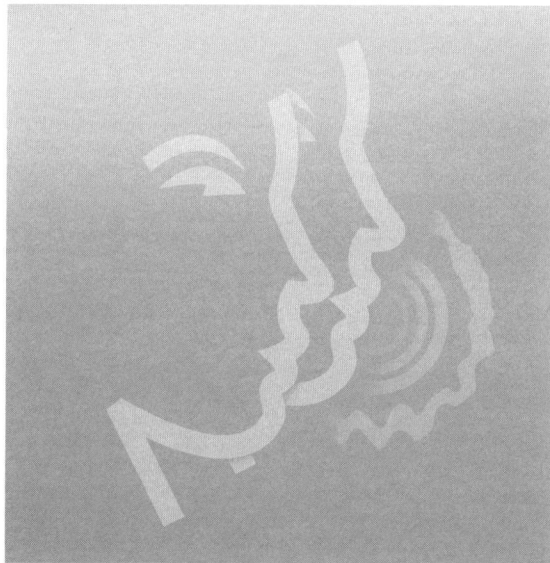

Jenny Hunt
& Alyson Slater

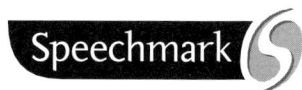

Speechmark (S

Speechmark Publishing Ltd
Telford Road, Bicester, Oxon OX26 4LQ, UK

Published by

Speechmark Publishing Ltd, Telford Road, Bicester, Oxon OX26 4LQ,
United Kingdom
Tel: +44 (0)1869 244644   Fax: +44 (0)1869 320040
www.speechmark.net

002-4758/Printed in the United Kingdom/1030

British Library Cataloguing in Publication Data
Hunt, Jenny
    Working with children's voice disorders. – (A Speechmark practical
    therapy manual)
    1. voice disorders – Treatment 2. Voice disorders in children
    3. Voice disorders in youth
    I. Title II. Slater, Alyson
    618.9'285506

ISBN 0 86388 279 X

Contents

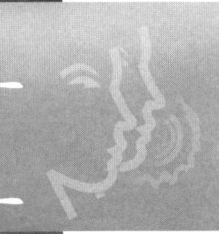

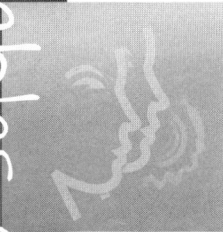

Tables and Figures

TABLES

FIGURES

Acknowledgements

We would like to acknowledge and thank our colleagues, whose enthusiasm for our initial articles and subsequent workshops on paediatric voice, persuaded us to 'have a go'. We are particularly grateful to Anne Somerville for showing Stephanie Martin our original Resource Pack; to Richard Todd for his patience and skill when all seemed lost (on the disc), and to John Pickles, Consultant Otolaryngologist, for his continuing support and referrals!

In addition, our heartfelt thanks goes to our families for their patience and support through every chapter, writer's block and crisis, real or imagined.

Foreword

At last, we have a basic yet comprehensive and user-friendly text that successfully combines the theory and practice of working with paediatric dysphonia. The authors share a wealth of ideas with us, and their approach makes the book recommended reading for any speech & language therapist working with dysphonia. I believe it will become a core text for students and clinicians, whether they are generalists or specialists in this field.

Hunt and Slater provide clear departmental standards of care; model case histories and clinical evaluation forms, and a voice care leaflet. I have found that many therapists do not gain much experience in working with dysphonic children, either because such children fail to get referred, or because they are treated in specialist centres. Having examples of the paperwork, which is so crucial these days, will save many readers the effort of 'reinventing the wheel'.

The authors raise key issues such as the appropriateness and timing of interventions, and do not allow the reader to fall into the trap of believing that dysphonia can only be due to vocal abuse. In fact, hoarseness can be a result of normal development.

This is an important book because the authors have addressed a significant gap in the market. I believe that therapists will be reassured and reinvigorated by using it; every department should have a copy.

Jayne Comins
Specialist Speech & Language Therapist (Voice)
Queen Elizabeth Hospital NHS Trust

Introduction

Working with Children's Voice Disorders has been written for speech & language therapists working with children in schools or community clinics, who have no specialist knowledge of voice. It is intended for clinicians who have limited numbers of this client group on their caseload, but who are committed to providing effective therapy to these children. It is also suitable for Speech and Language Therapy students.

The book begins with an overview of the development of the infant and juvenile larynges, highlighting the differences between the immature and mature structures, and the concomitant changes in voice. In designing an appropriate and realistic treatment programme, it is essential to take into account the nature of the voice problem. Therefore, the authors' next focus is on the contributory and maintaining factors of voice problems, setting the dysphonia into context. The authors guide the inexperienced therapist through taking a case history, and the assessment and evaluation of the child's voice, before discussing the principles of management with this potentially challenging client group.

The authors draw on over 10 years experience with children's voice disorders to give practical advice on therapy; the aims of intervention, and how best to achieve them. The later chapters contain practical ideas, therapy exercises, and forms for setting up groups, together with case studies and suggestions on how to evaluate therapy and measure outcomes.

The ideas suggested in this book work equally well in individual or group therapy settings, and it is hoped that they will give therapists the confidence and skills to take on children with voice disorders. This book is, in part, the authors' response to the pleas of colleagues over the years, such as 'I am seeing a six-year-old child with vocal nodules, HELP!'

Chapter 1: Laryngeal and Voice Development in Children

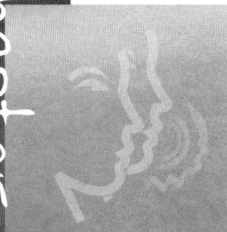

INTRODUCTION

The purpose of this chapter is to give a brief overview of the gross anatomical changes that occur within the larynx from infancy through to puberty, and the concomitant changes in voice. In order to appreciate the range of problems and contributory factors encountered when working with dysphonic children, it is essential to understand that the child's larynx is not a miniature version of the adult larynx. It is not the intention of the authors to go into detail on the function of the normal adult larynx, as this is well documented in other sources (Hirano *et al*, 1983; Mathieson, 2001; Martin & Lockhart, 2000). The focus in this chapter is on the processes of maturation, and how these are evident in the production of the young voice.

ANATOMICAL AND PHYSIOLOGICAL DEVELOPMENT: BIRTH TO PUBERTY

The Infant Larynx

The maturing of the structure of the vocal folds and the growth of the larynx are lengthy processes. As stated above, the child's larynx is not simply a miniature version of an adult larynx, but is an immature structure that is constantly changing.

The infant larynx differs from the adult's in terms of its position within the vocal tract, as well as in its size and shape, and structural maturity of its tissues. In the newborn, the larynx is situated high in the neck, and the pharyngeal cavity is short and lies horizontally, offering little resistance to airflow. This, together with the ability of the epiglottis to make contact with the soft palate, enables the infant to breathe while it feeds. The infant's airway is 'funnel-shaped', in contrast to the more 'tubular' shape of the adult's. This is the result of the growth of the cricoid cartilage, which widens the subglottic area (Figure 1).

No significant differences exist between male and female larynges in infancy, resulting in voices that are similar in both sexes. However, variance in size and weight of infants does influence laryngeal size. For example, pre-term babies may have considerably smaller larynges than full-term babies.

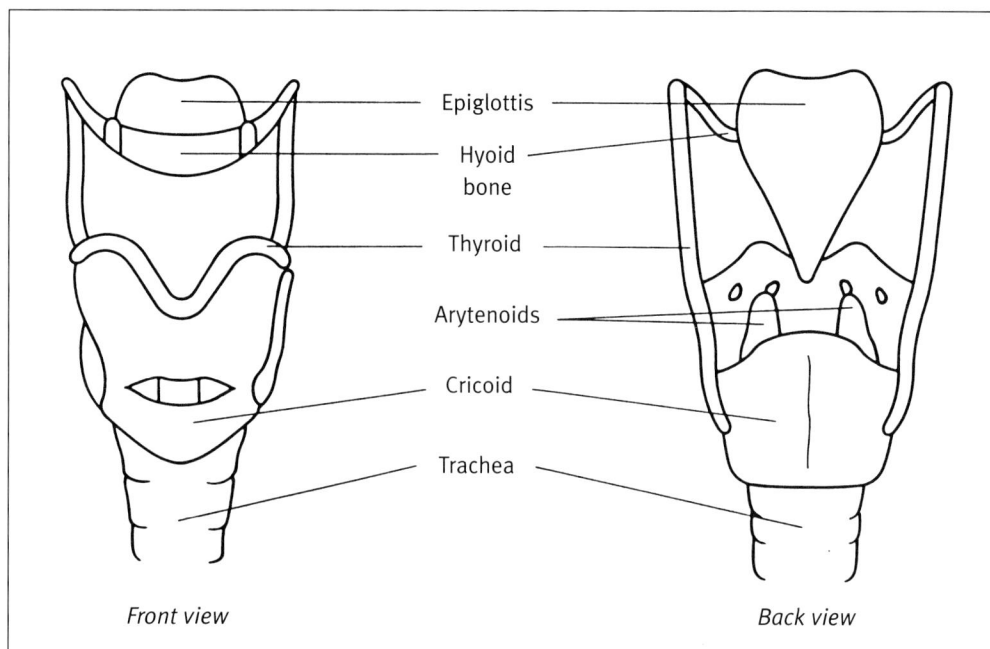

Figure 1
Cartilages of
the Larynx

Epiglottis

Hyoid
bone

Thyroid

Arytenoids

Cricoid

Trachea

Front view

Back view

There are various differences between the infant and adult larynx:

◆ In infancy, the laryngeal cartilages are both soft and pliable, with large
amounts of loose and highly vascular connective tissue. Thus the infant larynx
is more vulnerable than that of an adult and can easily become oedematous
following direct trauma, such as that following intubation.

◆ The infant thyroid cartilage is broader and shorter than the mature cartilage,
and this influences the shape of the larynx, making it more rounded than in
later life.

◆ The infant larynx is also more compact, with the cartilages assuming a large
proportion of the structure of the larynx (in particular the arytenoid
cartilages). As a result, the vocal folds are relatively short, producing a higher
fundamental frequency than the adult larynx. This is discussed in the second
part of this chapter.

◆ The infant vocal folds are morphologically immature. Hirano *et al* (1983) found
that the infant vocal folds not only lack mass, but also the physical properties
of the mature and sophisticated five-layered vibratory structure evident in
adulthood. Until this structure has fully developed, the immature vocal folds
are likely to be more vulnerable to vocal abuse (Figure 2).

Figure 2
Five-layered
Structure

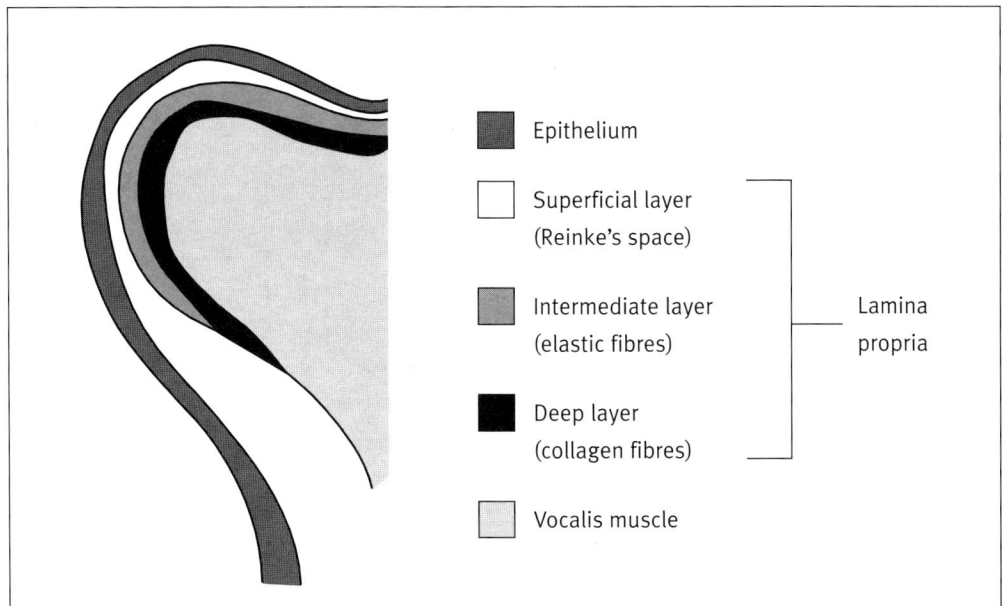

■	Epithelium
□	Superficial layer (Reinke's space)
▨	Intermediate layer (elastic fibres)
■	Deep layer (collagen fibres)
▨	Vocalis muscle

Lamina propria

Little is known about the neurological maturity of the infant larynx, but it has been suggested that this may not be fully developed until three years of age (Von Leden, 1985). Unfortunately, there is also little recent information on the intrinsic muscles of the infant larynx. However, a study by Kahane and Kahn (1984) found that the adductors (lateral cricoarytenoid; thyroarytenoid, and interarytenoid muscles) represented the bulk of the intrinsic muscle mass (Figure 3). It is speculated that functionally this relates to the muscles required to build up the intrathoracic and

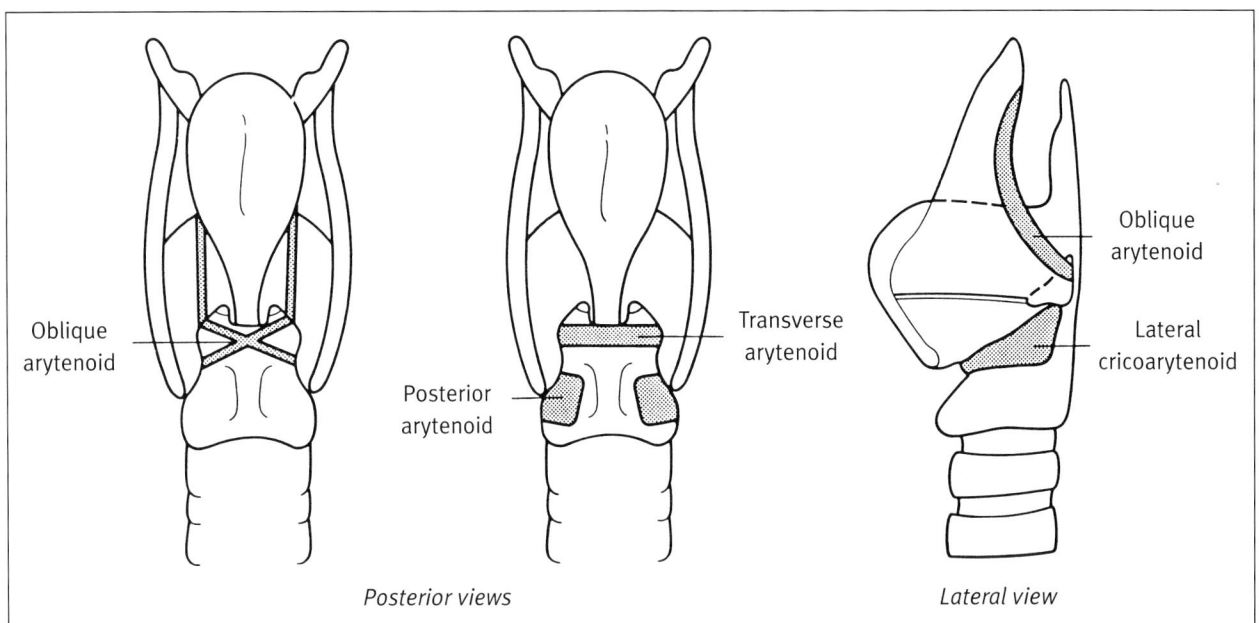

Oblique arytenoid

Posterior arytenoid

Transverse arytenoid

Oblique arytenoid

Lateral cricoarytenoid

Posterior views

Lateral view

Figure 3 Cross-sections of the Larynx Showing Intrinsic Muscles

intra-abdominal pressures necessary for the development of upper body strength, erect posture, walking, and the elimination of body waste. The cricothyroid muscle is the most massive muscle in the infant larynx, which may be attributable to adjustments needed during infant reflexive vocalisations and vocal play.

The Child Larynx

During childhood the position of the larynx changes. By the age of two years, it has descended from about C3–C4 to about C5. By five years, it has descended to C6. As a result, the pharynx increases in length, and by the age of five years it is no longer possible for the epiglottis to make contact with the soft palate. The shape of the vocal tract becomes more angulated and mature, and by the age of nine years its shape is comparable with that of an adult's, although it is obviously smaller in size.

The growth of the larynx and pharynx are correlated with growth in body height, and in childhood they remain the same for both sexes. Cartilages increase in size and firmness, and vocal folds increase in length. At four years old, the vocal folds – in particular the lamina propria – are poorly developed (Hirano, 1981; 1983). Although the fibrous connective tissues increase in density and structural complexity, these structures do not actually become 'mature' until after puberty. Boys' vocal folds grow at a greater rate than girls', being some 8 per cent larger by the age of nine years.

The Adolescent Larynx

As puberty approaches, the larynx begins to transform quite rapidly, and there is a sudden increase in the rate of growth. The larynx continues to descend in the neck, and by the end of puberty has reached its adult position at about C6–C7. It is during puberty that significant differences begin to emerge between the sexes.

By puberty, the male laryngeal cartilages are significantly larger and heavier than their female counterparts. The thyroid prominence is clearly more pronounced in males than females, and is typically referred to as the 'Adam's Apple'. Maddern *et al* (1991) believe this prominence is due to the change in angle of the thyroid cartilage, but this is disputed by Mathieson (2001).

Although growth of the larynx is associated with puberty in both males and females, antero-posterior growth in the male far exceeds that of the female. From pre-puberty to puberty, the male vocal folds undergo nearly twice as much growth as those of the female. The maturation of the lamina propria and vocal ligament continues in adolescence, and is not completed until after puberty. The change in the structural complexity of the vocal fold mucosa is a significant factor in voice change at puberty, as is the length of the vocal folds.

This maturation may be complete at about the age of 14 years in boys, but in girls it continues on average until about the age of 15–16 years. Pubertal growth of the larynx and of body height are closely related, and are obviously influenced by similar hormonal mechanisms.

The maturational changes that occur before and during puberty – that is, changes in length, width, thickness and biomechanical properties – result in significant changes in the adolescent voice, in particular the male voice. These will be discussed in more detail in the latter part of this chapter.

CHANGES IN VOCAL PARAMETERS AND NORM

When working with paediatric dysphonia, the clinician needs to remain aware of the maturation processes as well as the speed and constant nature of the changes.

The newborn infant arrives in the world with some innate skills, and the potential for developing an enormous range of further skills. One of the innate skills is the ability to respond positively to the human voice, most strongly its mother's.

Among the infant's host of potential skills lies the ability to communicate. It is the need to communicate that initiates the development of this defining human function. Throughout the development of communication, there is an intricate relationship between biological maturation processes, both physiological and neurological, and development prompted by acquisition of new knowledge and skills. Recent research (MacLarnon & Hewitt, 1999) suggests that modern humans and Neanderthals possess a larger thoracic vertebral canal than earlier hominids. This suggests a more highly developed channel, allowing innervation of the intercostal and abdominal muscles used to modify respiration during speech. This is one example of the evolutionary changes that have gone hand in hand with the development of speech in humans.

Respiratory Changes

The necessity for breathing exercises in adult voice work has been debated, and controversy exists over the role of breathing in voice therapy (Harris *et al*, 2000). Whichever school of thought the therapist follows, it is essential to remember that breathing is the power behind the production of voice. In children, the clinician should be aware that the development of phonic respiration begins at birth with the first cry. The crying baby is not automatically at risk of becoming dysphonic – on the contrary, crying is the first step towards the co-ordination of breathing with speech production.

During normal (vegetative) respiration, the length of inspiration equals that of expiration. The infant's first vocalisations at birth are the beginnings of later voluntary control of vegetative respiration. This ability to change the ratio of length of inspiration to length of expiration is essential for speech. It is this type of respiration that is known as phonic respiration. It has been postulated (Hunt & Slater, 1996) that the use of a dummy or pacifier in infancy that inhibits crying, may therefore restrict the development of phonic respiration.

Another factor affecting the development and refinement of phonic respiration is the change in volume of the rib cage, with a corresponding increase in lung size, during the second and third years of life (Boliek *et al*, 1997). Exercise increases the efficiency of the lungs, and is therefore also relevant to the development of phonic respiration. Much concern is currently centred on the increasingly sedentary lifestyle of children, and the implications this has for general fitness levels, as well as the risks of future heart disease. There are also implications for the development of efficient respiration, as a lack of exercise will reduce the development of the child's vital lung capacity. An adolescent's lung volume should be around four times that of a five-year-old (Mathieson, 2001). However, sedentary visual entertainment such as videos and playstations, and safety considerations due to such factors as increased road traffic and child abductions, have reduced traditional outdoor activities and physical exercise (Cotes, 1979) to the degree that the normal increase in lung volume may be impacted.

Vegetative Sounds

Crying is not the only sound produced by an infant: there are also burps, coughs and 'coos', which produce a response from the mother and other involved adults. These vegetative sounds reward the infant with a vocal response from the adult. The reinforcement of cooing usually takes the form of the adult imitating the infant's vocalisations. This process continues the development of phonic respiration. It is the precursor to the emergence of babble, because the interaction is so pleasurable for the baby that it continues to experiment with sounds.

Pre-verbal Communication

It is generally accepted that a mother knows the meaning of each of her baby's different cries. Research does not support this view (Mathieson 2001). It is also popularly believed that a mother can identify her own baby by its cry. Even before the individuality of the voice has been established, vocalisations are distinct in each infant. Pre-linguistic tonal development can occur from the age of two weeks (Mathieson, 2001). From this point an infant can produce melody, beginning with upward glides, and followed by rising and falling glides. By the time the infant is beginning to babble, at around three months, the wide range of frequencies in the babble increases the attractiveness of the sounds to adults, which in turn promotes positive reinforcement for the infant. The skill of using longer and more varied sound sequences has to be supported by a complementary skill in phonic respiration.

In these early months the infant has no ability to filter the sounds it hears, so all environmental sounds carry equal importance. The modern world is a noisy place to live in, and within the home there is often background noise such as TV, radio, or music, which means that the infant rarely experiences complete quiet. Any vocal input takes place against this level of background noise. The effects of this on language development are well documented (Ward & Birkett, 1992). Adult reinforcement of vegetative sounds, changes in frequency and babble will be 'lost' to the infant in the background noise. This will reduce the infant's output, and have a corresponding impact on the development of phonic respiration, language and speech skills.

Vocal Range

In the process of establishing a child's pitch, the fundamental frequency decreases until about the age of five years. For the first 141 days of life, a baby's cry has a fundamental frequency of 443 Hz for a boy and 414 Hz for a girl (Shephard & Lane, 1968). By the age of five years, the fundamental frequency for both sexes is around 254 Hz (White, 1995). Once established, the range of the voice is constant at about two and a half octaves for both boys and girls, and will remain so until the age of around 16 years. The singing range for boys and girls prior to puberty varies very little, and covers the middle octave.

Pitch at Puberty

The pubertal voice, with its accompanying pitch changes in adolescent boys, occurs as the larynx undergoes a period of rapid growth. The effect on the pitch of the young male's voice is a drop of around an octave. The rapidity of growth causes temporary losses of co-ordination of the muscles in the larynx, which are realised as the characteristic pitch breaks of the 'breaking' voice. The adolescent female also experiences changes in pitch associated with the growth of the larynx. However, these changes are not as extensive in girls as in boys, and they take place over a longer period of time. Therefore the 'breaking' voice is usually not as evident in girls, because control over co-ordination of the laryngeal muscles can be more easily maintained. The laryngeal changes are completed by the age of 15–16 years, whereas body growth continues for several more years.

SUMMARY

As stated at the beginning of this chapter, the immature larynx is a structure in a state of constant change. However, the structural and functional changes of the larynx cannot be viewed in isolation when working with the dysphonic child. It is important that these changes are set in context with the concurrent development of language and speech-production skills.

Chapter 2: The Origins of Paediatric Dysphonia

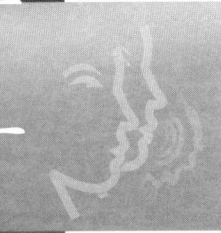

INTRODUCTION

In this chapter the complexity of dysphonia in children begins to emerge. There is a brief overview of the more common laryngeal disorders in children, and the likely involvement of a community speech & language therapist. The organic causes of dysphonia are usually a fairly small part of the overall picture. The majority of this chapter, therefore, is devoted to the wide array of other causal and maintaining factors. These factors may be divided into the following categories:

- Physical and developmental
- Medical
- Psychological and behavioural
- Cultural and environmental.

COMMON LARYNGEAL DISORDERS

Maddern *et al* (1991) describe laryngeal disorders under two categories – anatomical and neurological – and list 24 anatomical causes alone, which are further divided into three sub-groups: nose, oral cavity, pharynx; larynx; and tracheobronchial (Figure 4). It is true that there is a wide range of conditions that impact on voice. However, for the practising clinician, the more complex disorders are rare, and often bring with them a range of medical problems whose resolution is of greater importance for the child and family than any voice problem.

The authors believe that the clinician's skills are best focused where they can achieve maximum benefit to the child, and where the overriding clinical need is the resolution of a voice disorder. This usually encompasses the children presenting with vocal pathology such as nodules, laryngeal webs, polyps, or papilloma.

Incidence of Common Laryngeal Disorders

There is a paucity of recent research regarding the incidence of common laryngeal disorders in children. Miller and Madison (1984) found that 40 per cent of 249 children attending a voice clinic had vocal nodules, and of these 94 per cent were bilateral. Cornut and Troillet-Cornut (1995) support this, and found that 68 per cent of children identified as being dysphonic had nodular lesions. The remainder had

Figure 4
Anatomic
Difficulties
Associated with
Paediatric
Dysphonia

1 *Nose, Oral Cavity, Pharynx*
   Choanal atresia
   Micrognathia
   Pierre Robin syndrome
   Cleft Lip/Palate
   Tonsil and adenoid hypertrophy
   Macroglossia
   Ankyloglossia

2 *Larynx*
   Supraglottic
       Laryngomalacia
       Vallecular cyst
   Glottic
       Atresia, stenosis, cleft
       Laryngeal web
       Nodules, polyps, papilloma
   Subglottic
       Stenosis (acquired or congenital)
       Hemangioma

3 *Tracheobronchial*
   Stenosis (acquired or congenital)
   Tracheomalacia
   Extrinsic
       Congenital vascular anomaly
       Aberrant subclavian artery
       Aberrant innominate artery
       Vascular ring
       Mediastinal adenopathy/tumour
       Congenital goitre
   Intrinsic
       Foreign
       Granuloma

polyps, cysts or webs, and only 1.42 per cent had normal vocal cords. Pannbacker (1999) reported that the frequency of occurrence for vocal nodules in clinics is between 15 and 35 per cent, and Stone (1982) found them to exist more frequently in children than in adults.

The authors have run paediatric voice groups since 1991, and these have been attended mainly by children diagnosed as having vocal nodules. The development of assessment and diagnostic tools, such as videostroboscopy, in Joint Voice Clinics, has resulted in more accurate diagnoses. This means therapy can be targeted at children whose dysphonia can be remediated by therapy alone. The importance of an adequate diagnosis is discussed further in Chapter 3.

The high incidence of nodules has led some authors to question the validity of treatment. This debate will be examined in more detail in Chapter 4. Sander (1989) asked that clinicians be circumspect in treating childhood dysphonias, because he believed that the continual process of growth and maturation resulted in naturally occurring dysphonia. He further suggested that aurally skilled clinicians detect 'problems' that are within the normal range of vocal behaviours. Nonetheless, it is difficult to ignore the dysphonic child, especially one with vocal nodules, and hard to believe that a reliably functioning and good quality voice does not improve the child's ability to function as a social individual. The high incidence of nodules in itself should not suggest a state of 'normality', particularly when physiological changes have taken place.

As with all speech and language problems, the question of gender is also relevant. Miller and Madison (1984) found that out of 241 children having vocal nodules, thickened cords, oedematous cords and other pathologies, 162 were boys: that is, there were twice as many boys as girls.

This is reflected by the authors' experience, and is illustrated in Figure 5.

Research and the authors' experience clearly indicate that boys are more at risk of developing dysphonia than girls. This trend is reflected throughout the spectrum of communication problems, not just with voice. Although recent research seems to suggest a genetic link to speech and language problems, there is no hard evidence to support a similar link in the development of childhood dysphonia.

THE INVOLVEMENT OF OTHER COMMUNICATION PROBLEMS

It has already been stated that voice problems may co-exist with other problems that come within the remit of the speech & language therapist – for example, a cleft lip or palate. In this example, the imbalance of resonance needs to be dealt with in order to decrease the amount of work that the larynx undertakes as it attempts to counteract the resonance problem. The authors would always expect that the primary presenting problem should be addressed first.

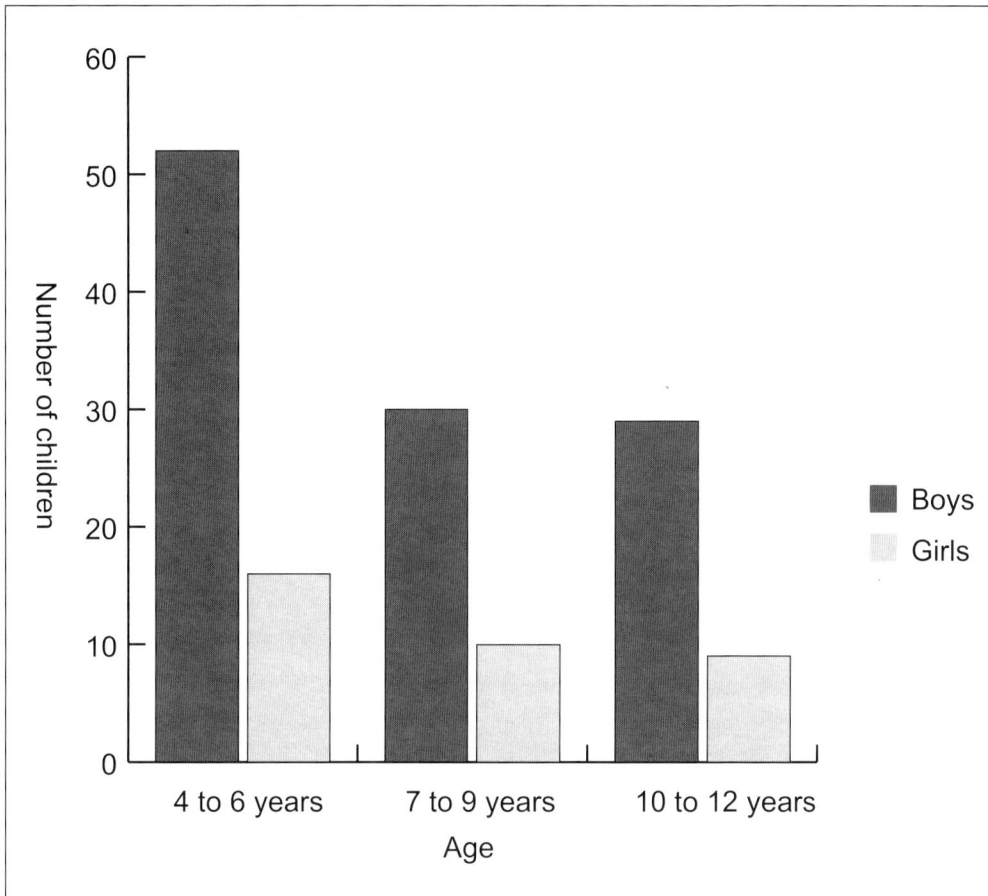

Figure 5
The Incidence of Dysphonia in Children Attending the Authors' Voice Groups (1991–1999)

Any language difficulties, whether they result from delay or disorder of acquisition, or from English being a second language, will cause the child to have difficulty in understanding some of the theories of the Voice Care Programme (covered in later chapters). In addition, the dysfluent child may have underlying problems that are manifesting themselves as either a dysfluency or a voice problem (Case Summaries 1 and 2, pp16–19). These may have to be addressed, or even referred to another agency, prior to successful therapy taking place.

Poor or ineffectual communication and social skills may have implications for the appropriateness of vocal behaviours in different environments or with different communication partners. If these skills are affected as a result of wider difficulties, such as autistic spectrum disorders, then the management of the dysphonia should be an integral part of the overall management of the child.

In conclusion, the clinician must decide which of the child's communication problems is primary, and whether or not the resolution of that problem will also resolve the voice problem.

CASE SUMMARY 1

Name:	Th
Age on Referral:	8,00
Initial Contact:	Referred by teacher for dysfluency. On assessment, he presented with mild dysfluency characterised by fluent initial sound repetition and occasional blocks. Th also presented with a hoarse voice, and was referred to the Voice Clinic.
Onset of Voice Problem:	Th's mother thought that his voice had always sounded 'gruff', and believed it to be normal for Th. His dysfluency had occurred sporadically for about two years.
Case History:	
Family:	Th was the third of four siblings, and had two brothers aged 11 and 13, and a six-year-old sister. There was no family history of dysfluency, or other speech or language problems.
Medical:	Th suffered from hay fever, and took antihistamine tablets in the summer months. At 19 months of age he was admitted to hospital for one night with a high temperature and a swelling on his neck caused by an infection. Th had a persistently blocked nose with excessive discharge, and suffered frequent ear infections. He snored, and his GP had noted enlarged tonsils.
Environment:	Th's father smoked in the home.
Behavioural:	Th's mother described him as very active, anxious and 'nervy'. He enjoyed karate, which he originally took up to increase his confidence. Th would often fight and argue with his sister and the brother closest to him in age.
Development:	Th was born at 34 weeks, but all milestones were within normal limits.
Posture:	Th was tall for his age, and tended to round his shoulders and carry his head forward.
Tension:	Excessive laryngeal tension.
Breathing:	Clavicular.
Voice Evaluation:	Moderately hoarse voice. Occasional phonation breaks. High pitch and narrow range.
Voice Clinic:	Tonsils large but clean, adenoids moderately large. Nose full of mucous. Large bilateral vocal nodules.

CASE SUMMARY 1 – CONTINUED

Management:

May 1991   Attended Children's Voice Group consisting of four hour-long sessions over four weeks. Th quickly grasped and implemented the Voice Care Programme. Voice quality improved and Th was placed on a six-month review.

September 1991   Review brought forward following contact from the family. Voice and fluency significantly worse since a local shopkeeper had mimicked Th's voice and dysfluency. Th attended a further set of groups in October 1991, and voice quality improved greatly; however, his dysfluency became more noticeable. This was discussed with Th and his family, who felt that further therapy could wait until the voice quality was well established.

January 1992   Th attended a further set of groups, as voice quality had not been maintained. In a quiet activity (drawing an animal the child would like to be) Th drew a bear 'to kill people who laugh at me'.

March 1992   At review, Th's mother believed that his voice quality and dysfluency varied directly in relation to problems at school, such as teasing and bullying. She felt that the family was able to manage Th's voice and dysfluency by dealing with issues that bothered him.

July 1992   At review, Th's dysfluency was severe, and he therefore attended an intensive dysfluency course consisting of four two-hour sessions in a week. Fluency improved, and Th felt more in control.

October 1992   At review, there was noticeable deterioration in both voice quality and fluency when discussing subjects Th did not like, such as a particular teacher at school. Th attended a further set of groups in January 1993, and achieved good voice and fluency.

September 1993   At review, voice quality was good, but Th's dysfluency was severe.

October 1993   Attended a further intensive dysfluency course.

February 1994   Both Th and his mother were very pleased with the maintenance of both voice quality and fluency.

May 1994   Fluency again causing concern, so Th attended an intensive dysfluency course in June 1994.

October 1994   At review, Th had a good quality voice and mild dysfluency, which he found acceptable.

April 1995   Review offered, but declined by the family, as there were no further concerns. Th was discharged, treatment complete aged 12,07.

CASE SUMMARY 2

Name:	D
Age on Referral:	2,10
Initial Contact:	Referred by the Health Visitor, who was concerned about poor language development. Advice was given to the family, and D's development was reviewed three times over a period of 11 months before the family were discharged for non-attendance.
Re-referral:	At chronological age 5,07, D was re-referred by his Headteacher for 'poor speech'. On assessment, D was noted as having reduced /s/ clusters, but the clinician was more concerned by D's voice quality, which was moderately hoarse.
Onset of Voice Problem:	D's mother had not noticed anything different about D's voice, and thought it was normal for him. She attributed the hoarseness detected by the clinician to a recent heavy cold. D was reviewed six weeks later, and a referral made to the Voice Clinic, as the voice quality remained poor.
Case History:	
Family:	D was the fourth child of eight, and had five brothers and two sisters, ranging in age from nine months to 12 years. There was a family history of dysfluency, delayed speech and language development, dyslexia and moderate learning difficulties.
Medical:	D had suffered from frequent ear infections in his first three years, but there was nothing else of note.
Environment:	Both parents smoked, although never in the same room as the children. Mother had a very relaxed style of parenting, and often had up to 14 children in the house at any one time.
Behavioural:	D was described as very energetic, noisy and extrovert, a child who was always chattering and could be heard above the rest.
Development:	D's developmental milestones were within normal limits.
Posture:	Shoulders slightly raised and head carried forward.
Tension:	Marked facial and laryngeal tension.
Breathing:	Clavicular.
Voice Evaluation:	Pitch appropriate, but narrow in range. Fast rate of speech and loud. Moderately hoarse.
Voice Clinic:	D's vocal folds were mildly congested and swollen, but there were no nodules.

CASE SUMMARY 2 – CONTINUED

Management: During a three-month period D was offered two Children's Voice Groups, each consisting of four hour-long sessions over four weeks. Attendance was sporadic and, although D was a responsive child who quickly learned the Voice Care Programme, there was no evidence of home support in implementing the Programme. D was discharged after failing to keep a review appointment.

Re-Referrals: At age 10,01, D was referred by the Special Educational Needs Co-ordinator teacher he was seeing in school. Concerns existed over D's voice and his behaviour. The family had also increased, with the birth of two additional sisters. Written advice was given to the family and school, and the family were invited to contact the clinician to discuss therapy options. Six months later, with no contact, D was discharged.

The Health Visitor in contact with the family referred D again at age 11,07, as his hoarse voice persisted and he was now dysfluent. He also had a diagnosis of severe emotional behavioural problems, and was attending a residential school. D was apparently most concerned by his dysfluency, so appointments to attend an intensive dysfluency group in half-term were sent. Unfortunately, D failed to attend or contact the department. He also failed to attend the next offered appointments for a dysfluency group, and was subsequently discharged.

A Community Paediatrician referred D at age 13,02, due to ongoing concerns about his voice and dysfluency. A re-referral to the Voice Clinic was made, and moderate bilateral nodules were diagnosed. In addition, a grommet was inserted in the left ear. D attended 10 individual sessions at his local clinic to improve his dysfluency and voice quality. As his voice quality improved, D decided he no longer wanted therapy and he was discharged, although a mild dysfluency persisted.

The child described in Case Summary 2 (pp 18–19) was later diagnosed as having behavioural problems and, as a result, voice therapy was unsuccessful. Voice therapy may only be successful where the voice problem exists in isolation.

CONTRIBUTORY AND MAINTAINING FACTORS

A child's voice is similar to an adult's, in that it reflects many aspects of their physical, cultural, social and psychological development, as well as being heavily influenced by the environment. These influences interweave with a great deal of complexity, and it is therefore important not to think of causal factors as simply a checklist to run through before arriving at a diagnosis.

It is too simplistic to attribute children's voice problems or the development of vocal nodules to 'vocally abusive behaviours', such as yelling, screaming, hard glottal onset, or speaking in noisy environments, or for prolonged periods of time. Most children participate regularly in these behaviours, and if such activities are the only factors responsible for nodule formation, it is surprising that more children, or indeed more adults, do not develop them. Many children yell, scream and strain their voices when playing, but remain free from vocal problems.

So, what is it, over and above this vocally abusive behaviour, that leads to the development of dysphonia in children, or to nodular formation? The probability remains that other elements contribute or pre-dispose certain children to the development of dysphonia. Table 1 summarises the factors contributing to the occurrence of dysphonia in children.

Physical and Developmental Factors

It has been well documented that the quality of voice is dependent on the structure of the vocal folds; the neuromuscular controls within the vocal apparatus, and vocal behaviour (Green, 1989; Schalen & Rydell, 1995). Dysphonia may result from abnormality of any of these factors. Given this commonly accepted understanding, it is likely that dysphonia in children may be partly attributable to the following physiological and developmental factors:

Table 1 Factors Contributing to the Occurrence of Dysphonia in Children			
Physical/ Developmental	**Medical**	**Psychological/ Behavioural**	**Cultural/ Environmental**
◆ Immature structure ◆ Inadequate respiratory patterns ◆ Dummies ◆ Excessive crying ◆ Lack of exercise ◆ Anatomical abnormalities	◆ Frequent upper respiratory tract infections ◆ Asthma ◆ Allergies ◆ Medication ◆ Hearing loss ◆ Cleft-palate ◆ Genetic factors ◆ Environmental irritants ◆ Gastro-oesophageal reflux	◆ Aggression ◆ Distractibility ◆ Disturbed peer relations ◆ Immaturity ◆ Exuberant/extrovert behaviour ◆ Tension/anxiety ◆ Frustration ◆ Attention-seeking and manipulative behaviour	◆ Communicative incompetence ◆ Shouting/ screaming ◆ Competition with noise ◆ Excessive use ◆ Singing ◆ Poor vocal models ◆ Imitation of peer group/TV characters ◆ Family dynamics ◆ Family size

◆ *Immature structure*

It is important to remember that the child's larynx is not just a miniature version of the adult larynx. As explained in Chapter 1, it is an immature and constantly changing structure. These age-related conditions of the gross anatomy of the vocal tract are responsible for several characteristics of the normal child's voice. These result in a voice that is lower in intensity, higher in pitch, smaller in range, and with more limited resonance than an adult's. It has been speculated that inappropriate vocal behaviour may be a result of the child's attempt to compensate for the immature voice pre-puberty, for example through strained phonation, or an inadequate increase in pitch (Schalen & Rydell, 1995).
The gradual development of the vocal ligament; the maturation of the vocal muscles, and the continuous increase of the phonatory/respiratory glottis ratio (Hirano, 1991) all exert modulatory effects on glottal function until after puberty. Hence the immature morphology of the vocal folds may perhaps explain the child's increased susceptibility to microtraumatic lesions and the occurrence of nodules.

◆ *Inadequate respiratory patterns*

Persistent or recurrent alterations in the respiratory structures may predispose a child to adopt compensatory vocal behaviours. It is important to note any history of respiratory distress following birth, or any prolonged periods of intubation, which may not only have altered respiratory patterns, but also have resulted in direct trauma to the vocal folds themselves. Following a premature birth, uncoordinated muscle activity (especially during sleep) may give rise to aberrant respiratory patterns. The thoracic muscles may try to inspire while the abdominal muscles expire (West, 1979). These poor respiratory patterns may be accompanied by excessive laryngeal tension as the child attempts to compensate.

◆ *Dummies or Pacifiers*

It is possible that children who are given dummies to pacify prolonged or excessive crying may ultimately be at risk of developing dysphonia. As discussed in Chapter 1, crying provides essential preliminary exercise for phonic respiration, allowing the development of efficient respiratory patterns. If this is suppressed with the use of a dummy or pacifier, then the child is unable to practise such preliminary exercises.

◆ *Excessive crying*

On the contrary, however, it has also been documented that prolonged crying as a baby may lead to the development of vocal nodules (Greene, 1980). In the authors' experience, there does not appear to be a strong link between prolonged crying or screaming and the development of vocal nodules. Most new babies spend a considerable amount of time crying, which does not appear to affect them in any way – only the parents!

◆ *Lack of exercise*

Children who do not exercise regularly may be more vulnerable to dysphonia as the lack of exercise affects the size of the lungs, which ultimately may affect airflow and phonation (Cotes, 1979). These findings may reflect the authors' observation of an increase in the incidence of dysphonia in children over the last 15 years, as lifestyles have become more sedentary with an increase in the use of cars, computer games and television. Prolonged sitting may also give rise to postural changes such as an anterior head position, which may have a direct effect on tensions in and around the vocal tract.

◆ *Anatomical abnormalities*

It is worth mentioning that anatomical difficulties or abnormalities within the vocal tract may contribute to the development of dysphonia in children. As previously mentioned, this book will not dwell on voice problems that are the result of gross abnormalities, for example Pierre Robin syndrome.

Medical factors

Alterations that occur in the vocal tract as a result of medical conditions can heighten a child's susceptibility to dysphonia. Conditions that occur repeatedly, or that result in compensations that are habituated across time, are significant in precipitating voice problems. These include:

◆ *Frequent upper respiratory tract infections*

All children suffer from Upper Respiratory Tract Infections (URTIs) at some time or another. It is possible that the children who are more at risk of developing dysphonia are those who frequently suffer from URTIs that give rise to an acute laryngitis (acute inflammatory condition). The child has no time to recover between each episode. This leads to regular mouth-breathing, resulting in a drying out of the vocal folds, coughing, and constant throat clearing. Infected post-nasal discharge may also act as an irritant, as evidenced by the children described in Case Summaries 1 (pp 16–17) and 3 (p24). There may also be a general reduction in oral and/or nasal resonance, with the resulting imbalance leading to strain at the laryngeal level as the child struggles to gain quality, volume and power.

◆ *Asthma*

Children who suffer from asthma may have periodic partial occlusion of the airway that affects their airflow during phonation. It is quite common to see fairly aberrant breathing patterns in asthmatic children. These may ultimately give rise to excessive laryngeal tension as the child attempts to compensate. Incessant coughing during asthma attacks may lead to vocal abuse. Any condition of the upper respiratory tract that produces excessive secretions resulting in coughing and throat-clearing will predispose the child to vocal abuse, because of the vigorous approximation of the vocal folds. In addition,

CASE SUMMARY 3

Name: R

Age on Referral: 5,02

Initial Contact: Referred by the GP for a 'husky catch in his voice' and a query as to whether 'his soft palate is functioning entirely normally or if he is failing to use it to best effect'.

Onset of Voice Problem: R's mother had noticed that his voice had grown husky since starting school. She felt that he was doing too much singing.

Case History:

Family: R was the eldest of two children, and had a three-year-old sister. There were no other speech or language concerns, and no significant family history.

Medical: R did not have any allergies, but he had a history of URTIs for which the GP usually prescribed antibiotics. Mother reported that R was very prone to coughs and colds, and was a persistent throat-clearer.

Environment: The family lived in a centrally heated home, where neither parent smoked. R enjoyed spicy food.

Behavioural: R's mother described him as a shy little boy who was a chatterbox at home, but who did not particularly shout. He enjoyed singing.

Development: All milestones were within normal limits.

Posture: No problems noted.

Tension: Moderate laryngeal tension.

Breathing: Clavicular.

Voice Evaluation: Fast rate of speech, and loud. Breathy phonation. Occasional phonation breaks.

Voice Clinic: Enlarged adenoids and tonsils. Direct laryngoscopy showed small bilateral nodules.

Management: During an eight-month period, R attended five sets of Children's Voice Groups, each set consisting of four hour-long sessions over four weeks. Within each session R would demonstrate an improved quality of voice, which was not maintained between sessions. Any work sent home was not completed. Initially R was a quiet group member, but he gradually became more mischievous and disrupted the sessions.

It was decided to make the family involvement more direct, and R was offered five individual sessions, which built upon the work done in the groups. His mother remained in the room, and specific activities to do at home were given following each appointment. A 'contract' was agreed between the clinician, R and his mother, in which the clinician would demonstrate how to improve voice quality, and R and his mother would do the work at home.

Voice quality was maintained fairly well over a three-month review. A further three individual sessions were offered, followed by a six-month review, after which R was discharged.

incorrect use of inhalers can deposit the medication on the vocal folds rather than in the lungs, and act as an irritant.

◆ *Allergies*

Children who experience frequent allergic reactions may be at risk of dysphonia, especially if their lifestyle includes many activities that are vocally demanding. Allergies lead to congested mucous membranes; as a result, the voice lacks nasal resonance, and the quality may be breathy. Normal reflexive activities such as sneezing and coughing, if they occur repeatedly because of irritation or congestion, may also become habituated and result in abuse to the vocal mechanism. Wilson (1987) found a family history of allergy in about 25 per cent of children with laryngeal dysfunction. Allergic rhinitis afflicts more people than any other kind of allergic reaction, and is typically caused by airborne allergens.

◆ *Medication*

Some medications may significantly affect vocal tract function – for example, antihistamines may lead to a general drying out of mucosal membranes and thickening of mucosal secretions. In addition, bronchodilators commonly used in the treatment of asthma can cause irritation to the vocal folds.

◆ *Hearing loss*

A hearing loss may give rise to problems with auditory discrimination. As a result, the child may habitually use voice with great intensity and put an obvious strain on the vocal mechanism.

◆ *Cleft palate*

The presence of a cleft palate may give rise to an obvious imbalance of resonance, leaving the larynx to work harder in order to compensate. The child uses excessive force in order to try to maintain an adequate oral airstream. In addition, where velopharyngeal closure is not possible due to the extent of the cleft, closure is achieved at the level of the glottis. Furthermore, the intelligibility of children with a cleft palate is reduced. It is therefore quite common among this group of children for secondary vocal strain to occur.

◆ *Genetic factors*

Schalen and Rydell (1995) state that susceptibility to infectious or immunological injury of the vocal fold mucosa caused by genetically predisposing factors needs to be considered in the development of vocal nodules. It seems possible that genetic defects of molecular components may predispose towards chronic lesions of the vocal folds.

◆ *Environmental irritants*

These are more obvious in terms of contributory factors. Most therapists understand the effects of irritants on the vocal cord mucosa. Smokey or dry atmospheres, dust, fumes and fur may all contribute to the development of dysphonia in children.

◆ *Gastro-oesophageal reflux*

There has been more written about the effects of acid reflux in adults with dysphonia than in children, but it is worth noting its place in the development of dysphonia in children. Niedzielska *et al* (2000) confirmed that, on clinical assessment, children with gastro-oesophageal disease presented with inflammatory lesions in the posterior part of the larynx, as well as pathological changes in voice acoustic tests.

Pyschological and Behavioural Factors

The presence of vocal nodules in children has traditionally conjured up a mental picture of vocal abuse in the 'vociferous' child. Green (1989) suggests that such a focus is too simplistic, and that therapists working with a child with nodules may need to consider a multiplicity of psychological and behavioural variables. For example, an alternative personality type could be the shy, sensitive child, who often appears to be tense due to underlying anxieties (see Case Summary 4, pp27–28).

The behavioural characteristics of children with vocal nodules have been shown to include a predilection towards aggression, distractibility, disturbed peer relations, and immaturity (Green, 1989). Vocally abusive behaviours may appear in the child who is exuberant and extroverted, or in the tense, angry, frustrated child, who uses their voice as a means of expressing negative emotions (Mathieson, 2001). An

CASE SUMMARY 4

Name:	K
Age on Referral:	6,03

Initial contact: Due to her mother's concern, K was referred to ENT by her GP, as she had been suffering from a hoarse voice for four to five weeks. K was diagnosed with chronic laryngitis and congested vocal folds, and an adenotonsillectomy was recommended. There was a small unilateral nodule on the right vocal fold. The Consultant also referred to Speech and Language Therapy.

Onset of Voice Problem: K had experienced bouts of hoarseness for as long as her mother could remember, but the hoarseness had become continuous over the previous four months. This coincided with the birth of her younger sister. Her mother had always felt that the hoarseness was due to K's love of singing.

Case History:

Family: K was the middle of three sisters, the others being aged eight years and three months. There were no other speech or language concerns, and no relevant family history.

Medical: Frequent URTIs. Medication to help K to sleep (see *Behavioural*).

Environment: There were no smokers in the family. K was reported to have a good fluid intake.

Behavioural: K was a very highly strung little girl. She exhibited excessive tension in the assessment, constantly wringing her fingers. She had stopped eating prior to her sixth birthday, as a girl at school had said she was fat. This was manifestly untrue. The family had dealt with this, and resolved the issue. K had persistent dreams concerning a man in her bedroom, and her GP had prescribed medication to help her sleep and was monitoring the situation. Following a recent school topic on the dangers of talking to strangers, K had become convinced that a strange man was hiding in the garden shed. She would run indoors if a stranger walked past the end of the drive. Her mother described her as very sensitive and shy, although a bit of a comedienne within the family. K was aware of her voice, and that it deteriorated during the day.

Development: Normal development.

Posture: Characteristically hunched, with raised, rounded shoulders.

Tension: Marked tension in upper body, and particularly the face, neck and shoulders.

Breathing: Clavicular.

Voice Evaluation: Pitch high, but able to use a normal range. Fast rate of speech. Voice strained. Moderately dysphonic.

Management: *October 1992*   Attended four hour-long group sessions over a four-week period. She was well-motivated, and quickly implemented skills covered in group sessions. A lot of support was given in using the Voice Care Programme at home.

January 1993   Following a three-month review, K had maintained a good voice quality until the Christmas holidays. She attended two further groups in February and April 1993, and was put on a six-month review to try to maintain her voice quality improvement.

Voice Clinic: *April 1993*   Removal of vocal nodule.

Management: *October 1993*   On review K was mildly dysphonic, and she attended a set of group sessions in November 1993. Her mother was concerned that her school was not supporting the Voice Care Programme. The clinician contacted school and reinforced the importance of supporting therapy. K was placed on a six-month review. At age 7,05, K displayed a great deal of insight and self-awareness.

May 1994   Voice quality maintained, apart from a brief period of hoarseness following some bullying at school and the theft of the family car. School and home had dealt with this, and K and her mother felt confident in managing voice quality. A further six-month review was agreed.

November 1994   At review, K was discharged, her treatment complete. She was discharged from the Voice Clinic the following month.

example of such a child is outlined in Case Summary 2 (pp18–19). Also, if children get what they want when they talk loudly or use a 'whining' tone, or they keep talking incessantly, they learn to perpetuate those vocal strategies.

Bagnell (1982) suggests that children with nodules have difficulties verbalising intense emotions, so they vent their frustration and anger by screaming during play, in an attempt to develop an emotional vocabulary and manipulate child–parent relationships. Bagnell went on to suggest that such children display other manifestations of emotional inadequacy and parental manipulation, such as insensitivity to instructional control, an absence of turn-taking, and hyperactivity.

Cultural and Environmental Factors

Shouting, screaming and overuse

It has already been said that it is too simplistic to attribute children's vocal nodules to shouting and over-use. If it is assumed that this is typical vocal behaviour by young children, then any factors that reinforce this existing tendency must be looked at.

If one considers modern childhood, it is not hard to recognise a significant trend of vocal abuse. To look initially at entertainment for children, it is clear that vocal abuse is not only necessary, but is also positively encouraged, and is seen as the most definitive sign of a child's delight. From 'Crackerjack' in the 1960s/1970s to the present day, most television programmes for children set in place ritualised chants or vocal encouragement to game contestants – for example '50:50'. Even in Punch and Judy, a venerable form of entertainment, the child is required to participate vocally.

Many small children become involved in after-school clubs and activities where group participation is measured by the amount of shouting and screaming. There are also team sports – for example, football – demanding not only shouting by the spectators, but also between team players, usually in cold weather.

Cultural factors can include religious activities such as chanting of verses from the Koran in the Mosque. In the authors' experience, there is a higher percentage of Muslim boys presenting with vocal nodules than would be expected from the population (Jones *et al*, nd).

Singing

Children usually participate in singing in school, whether as part of an assembly, or in a lesson or choir. It is rare that teachers conducting such a lesson have any training in voice production or singing. What is common though, is the exhortation to children to 'open their mouths' and 'sing up'. The former can create an adverse posture for the larynx, while the latter encourages the forced production of voice.

Parent/carer and peer model

All therapists working with children are aware of the need to view the child both holistically, and within contexts such as the family or school. Parents influence early vocal behaviour, initially through the child imitating their voice; later, the peer group assumes greater significance. The development of the child's voice is affected by their experimentation with vocal strategies, and the patterns of reinforcement operating in the home and school environment. In some children, imitation of poor vocal models and a faulty learning technique may contribute to the development of a voice problem.

Family size and dynamics

This may be quite a significant factor in the development of dysphonia in ethnic minority children (Jones *et al*, nd). The family is often large and extended, the younger child (often the one presenting with dysphonia) may compete for attention, and siblings may also provide a constant source of confrontation. Both of these factors are evident in Case Summary 5 (pp31–32). Case history information such as the size and dynamics of a family are essential if therapy is going to be targeted within a realistic framework.

SUMMARY

It is clear that deviant vocal behaviour cannot be considered in isolation. Children with dysphonia are using their voices in a particular way, and this response pattern may be the result of the interplay between anatomical, physiological, social, emotional and environmental factors. These children are operating within a variety of contexts, and these contexts all need to be considered.

CASE SUMMARY 5

Name: T

Age on referral: 6,06

Initial Contact: T was referred to the Voice Clinic by his GP following concerns from his father that T's voice was 'husky'.

Onset of Voice Problem: The family believed that T's voice had been 'strained' from around the age of four years. This had been accepted as being normal for T until family friends had passed comments.

Voice Clinic: Moderate bilateral nodules.

Case History:

Family: T was the fifth of seven children, with sisters aged 15, 12 and eight years, and brothers aged nine and four years (twins).

Medical: T suffered frequent chest infections, but there was no history of allergies or hearing loss. T was a persistent throat-clearer.

Environmental: Father smoked, and the family liked to eat spicy foods. T did not have a very high fluid intake, but did drink cola straight from the fridge.

Behavioural: T was described as extrovert and 'always on the go'. He was known in the family as the most talkative and a shouter.

Development: Development was within normal limits for his age, but T was experiencing some learning difficulties at school. He had only been exposed to English from the age of four.

Posture: T was small for his age and tended to carry his shoulders slightly raised.

Tension: Marked laryngeal tension.

Breathing: Clavicular.

Voice Evaluation: Pitch high and narrow in range. Severe dysphonia and periods of aphonia. Voice hoarse and strained.

Management: *February–April 1993*   T attended two Children's Voice Groups, each consisting of four hour-long sessions over four weeks. There was good home support, and T learned the theory of voice care, but there was little or no implementation. In view of his relatively limited English and his slight learning difficulties, it was agreed with his father that a six-month review period was appropriate, to allow for maturation.

October 1993   T was reviewed in the Voice Clinic and the Consultant decided to remove the nodules (December 1993). The family reported that T was told not to use his voice for one week post surgery. He was discharged after two days, and began shouting as soon as he returned home.

February 1994   Voice Clinic review, re-referred to Children's Voice Group as again severely dysphonic.

CASE SUMMARY 5 – CONTINUED

March–May 1994   Attended two further sets of groups. T enjoyed these immensely, and began to be the group joker. The clinician visited T's school and discussed implementing a Programme of Voice Care with the Special Needs teacher.

August 1994   T attended a further four group sessions, and managed to achieve an improvement in voice quality within each session. However, the clinicians and T's father agreed that he was poorly motivated and needed further maturation. T's father agreed to contact the clinic.

May 1995   T reviewed following family contact. Three individual sessions followed by a set of four group sessions improved his voice quality greatly. A four-month review was agreed to trial maintenance of voice quality.

February 1996   At review, T's voice quality was moderately dysphonic. Unfortunately, the family failed to attend any appointments offered and T was discharged from the clinic.

Voice Clinic: *December 1996*   Reviewed by the Consultant and re-referred back to the Children's Voice Group.

Management: Attended two sets of groups in April and May 1997, but without motivation. Discharged in August 1997 after failing to keep a review appointment.

Voice Clinic: *December 1997*   Reviewed and re-referred to Children's Voice Group.

Management: *March–November 1998*   Attended a set of four groups, and then the clinician and T's father agreed to manage the Voice Care Programme at home, with support from the clinician via telephone and individual appointments as requested by the family. When implementing skills learned in therapy, T was able to achieve a good voice quality, but he was unable to maintain this.

January 1999   Following a review at the Voice Clinic, which showed that the nodules had disappeared, it was again discussed with T that he was responsible for his voice quality. At the age of 12,07 T's voice was harsh and strained. He remained small for his age, with persisting learning difficulties, and was not at all concerned about his voice. He was discharged from the clinic.

Chapter 3: Assessment and Evaluation

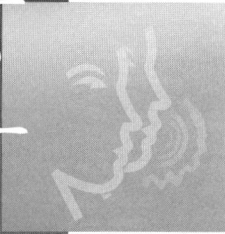

INTRODUCTION

The key to successful evaluation of a child's voice lies in the ability to unravel some of the complexities described in Chapter 2, as well as being able to interpret the visual, kinaesthetic and acoustic components of vocal behaviour. Ideally, the speech & language therapist needs to be both a specialist in voice disorders and a specialist in paediatrics. This is rarely the case, so any clinician attempting to assess a child's voice needs to acquire sound knowledge of the developmental process, including an awareness of the immature larynx, as well as an understanding of the child's communicative and cognitive level.

This chapter describes how to take a paediatric voice case history, and then looks at assessment procedures carried out by the speech & language therapist in clinic. There is also reference to the importance of assessing a child within a voice clinic setting.

TAKING A PAEDIATRIC VOICE CASE HISTORY

The case history is a collection of information that is critical to the evaluation and treatment of a voice disorder. The intention behind a case history is to learn more about the child's physical and emotional wellbeing, to identify any medical conditions that are likely to contribute to the dysphonia, and finally to look at their lifestyle and vocal demands.

There are many good books that cover the subject of taking a case history with voice patients (Martin & Lockhart, 2000; Colton & Casper, 1990; Mathieson, 2001), and they document various forms and checklists. There are far fewer that document the process of taking a voice case history in a child (Boone, 1980; Andrews, 1999). The aim of this chapter, therefore, is to highlight the areas that need to be addressed with children, as well as stressing the role that the family has to play.

Gathering Information

Unlike the adult with dysphonia, case history information is usually gained from either the parent or guardian, although in older children it can be extremely beneficial to seek out some of this information from the child. The clinician is able to gain insight into the child's level of awareness of the voice problem; perhaps to begin to discuss some feelings relating to their voice and, more obviously, to begin to build up a therapeutic relationship with the child.

Case history information is usually best achieved via an interview with the parent or guardian. A case history questionnaire can be completed by the parent or guardian prior to the initial assessment, but it is imperative that this is discussed fully during the initial assessment, and not seen purely as a 'time-saver'.

The authors have devised a specific Paediatric Case History Form (Appendix 1) to enable clinicians to elicit the information; however, it is important not to think of this as simply a checklist to run through before arriving at a diagnosis. It will form the basis of, and underpin, an appropriate management plan for the child, ensuring that any therapy is targeted within a realistic framework.

Some clinicians prefer to interview the parent or guardian separately from the child, and if two clinicians are available this would be the preferred option. While one clinician interviews the parent or guardian and takes a case history, the other begins to build up a rapport with the child prior to assessment. Once the child is relaxed, the same clinician can go on to assess their voice. Alternatively, it can be valuable if the child remains in the room playing while the interview takes place. The child may be more relaxed and, while playing on their own, may produce far more natural voice for the clinician to observe. The clinician also gains insight into the use of the voice while playing and interacting with the parent or guardian and, in addition, witnesses at first hand how the child uses their voice to attract the attention of others!

Onset and History of the Voice Problem

It can be quite difficult for parents to remember specific details about the onset of their child's voice problem, with replies such as 'his voice has been like this as long as I can remember', or 'he has been like this since he began to talk'. It is therefore imperative that the clinician asks more specific questions to allow the parent to explore this a little further. It is more difficult if the onset has been gradual, and this alone may give the clinician vital information about the likely contributory factors.

For example, children who move from one URTI into another, with reduced nasal airway as a result, will quickly develop patterns of misuse as they try to compensate. The consequent changes to the voice may appear gradually over time.

If the parent or guardian reports that the onset of the voice problem has been sudden, the clinician needs to explore precipitating factors such as traumatic injury as a result of vocal abuse. Medical problems preceding voice change in the child need to be explored (it is not uncommon for a granuloma to occur after intubation, for example). The clinician also needs to investigate any change in the child's environment prior to the onset, which may have led to an increase in muscular skeletal tension.

Variations in the child's voice quality are often difficult for the parent or guardian to describe. Voice quality descriptions are still a major source of controversy for the so-called 'experts', let alone the parent without knowledge or expertise. Words such as 'squeaky', 'rough', or 'sounds like he has a sore throat', can be used to enable the parent to answer some of the questions relating to the child's voice quality. Comparatives such as higher or lower enable a parent to think about and describe their child's pitch. The clinician needs to find out whether or not the child's voice is the same at home and at school. Is it worse towards the end of a day, or is it worse first thing in the morning? The latter is of significance if the child is also coughing and frequently clearing their throat, as this may indicate that they are suffering from some gastro-oesophageal reflux. If the child is old enough, and has some insight, it is worth asking them about sensory symptoms such as dryness, pain, soreness, ache or discomfort. Descriptive words such as these provide the clinician with essential diagnostic information.

The clinician needs to discuss the effect of the voice problem on the child and the family. This is the beginning of one of the most important considerations in working with paediatric dysphonia; it is not just the voice problem within the child that is being managed, but the way the child is interacting within their environment. 'Voice is a barometer of physical and emotional health and a bridge between the child and her world' (Andrews, 2001).

Voice Use and Vocal Demands

As the clinician takes the parent or guardian through the case history, a picture is formed of the child within their environment. Questions need to be asked about the child's voice use at home and with any siblings. It is not sufficient simply to ask whether or not the child shouts a lot (a common question asked by otolaryngology colleagues!), because as suggested earlier in this book, all children shout, and therefore other factors need to be explored:

◆ Does the child talk incessantly?

◆ Can they vary their voice according to the situation – for example, in the library?

◆ How many siblings are there, and what is the child's position in the family? The child may use their voice to compete with their siblings.

◆ How does the child use their voice at school? It is worth asking the parent or guardian if a teacher has made any comments about how the child uses their voice in the classroom or during PE. A telephone conversation with the child's teacher may add valuable information.

◆ What other vocal activities is the child involved in? The clinician needs to find out about any extra vocal activities that the child is involved with – for example, singing, drama, choir, sports or strenuous exercise. The latter, for instance, encourages a forceful closure of the glottis that puts a strain on the vocal apparatus, particularly if the child is using the voice at the same time.

◆ How much vocal flexibility does the child have? For example, how well does the child use their voice over noise? Children with dysphonia will often have limited vocal options, and therefore the only way they know to change any aspect of their voice is to increase the vocal effort, which often results in increased laryngeal tension.

Although most people are thrown by questions relating to personality, if the clinician is careful in their wording, they can begin to gain a picture of the child's personality type. Again, the clinician can use comparative words such as quiet or noisy, shy or confident. Most parents, once prompted, will talk happily about their offspring for hours! Important questions to ask might include, 'How does he/she gain your attention?' or 'Do they whine or talk incessantly?' These kinds of questions will tell the clinician a lot about possible patterns of misuse.

Family

In the authors' experience it is not uncommon to discover, when taking the case history, that there are one or more members of the family with either a reported voice disorder or similar voice quality. The authors have come across whole families with vocal nodules, for example, and this is often not just the children, but one of the parents too. This supports the theory, mentioned in Chapter 2, that children learn patterns of vocal behaviour that can contribute to vocal misuse from their parents as well as their peers.

This is usually an appropriate time to begin to explore carefully whether the child is under any degree of stress at home or at school. However, when asking these kinds of questions, it is essential that the clinician explains the relationship between stress and the voice, as well as the effect of any increase in muscular skeletal tension on the laryngeal musculature. The clinician needs to handle this kind of question sensitively, and to stress that the family are in no way to blame for the onset of the dysphonia.

Significant Medical History

Clinicians working in paediatrics will be more than competent to take down details regarding to a child's developmental milestones, so we will not dwell on this subject long. It is necessary to say, however, that the clinician will still need to explain why they are asking these questions in relation to the voice disorder. A birth history is vital to ascertain any possible trauma to the vocal apparatus. Questions need to be asked about any respiratory problems following the birth; periods of intubation, or feeding problems as a neonate. Medical problems such as asthma, allergies, frequent coughs or colds and URTIs need to be included, and whether or not the child is a mouth-breather, as this will dry out the vocal folds. Some medication will result in drying out of the vocal tract, and poor use of inhalers can lead to the medication 'sitting' on the vocal folds themselves, causing irritation, as mentioned in Chapter 2.

It is vital to know whether or not the child has any degree of hearing loss, because this will affect their ability to monitor their own voice, in particular the ability to adjust their volume. Even children with intermittent problems, such as glue ear, may find it difficult to monitor and therefore adjust their volume. The persistent use of a slightly increased volume may lead to some vocal misuse.

Irritants and Environmental Factors

Any factor that results in the drying out of the vocal folds must be noted, because it will lead to throat irritation and frequent coughing. It is worth asking the parent or guardian about the child's levels of hydration, and in particular what they like to drink. Cola, for example, contains caffeine, which is a diuretic and can also result in dehydration and subsequent irritation to the vocal folds. In addition, the clinician should note the amount of fluid drunk during a typical day.

Irritant factors also include dry or dusty atmospheres, central heating, spicy foods, hay fever and allergies. The results of these have already been discussed in Chapter 2. Even though the clinician is taking a case history for a child, it is worth remembering to ask specifically about whether or not the child is exposed to cigarette smoke. This must be handled sensitively, as it would be easy for parents or guardians who smoke to begin to blame themselves for their child's voice problem. The clinician must explain the negative effects of smoking on the vocal folds; however, they must also make sure that the parents are aware that although this may be a contributory factor, it is by no means the sole cause of the dysphonia.

Throughout the taking of the case history, the clinician must ensure that their questioning does not increase parental anxiety, as this will only lead to tension within the family unit. By the end of the session, parents should have an understanding of what may have contributed towards their child's voice problem, and therefore what needs to be done in order to make some changes in vocal behaviours, the child's environment and their lifestyle.

VOICE EVALUATION AND ASSESSMENT

The first part of this chapter has focused on the diagnostic information gleaned through taking a case history, which is a crucial first step in designing an appropriate and realistic programme of management. Once this has been achieved, the clinician needs to begin to evaluate the characteristics of the voice disorder, in order to determine the relative efficacy of various treatment approaches. The latter assessment will also be essential in order to formulate a prognosis.

The authors intend to concentrate on the perceptual evaluation of the child's voice, rather than assessment with the use of instruments. In Mathieson (2001) there is a comprehensive description of this kind of acoustic analysis, which would enable clinicians to gain a fuller understanding of the type of instrumentation and the acoustic parameters. The reality of the clinic situation, especially when working with children, usually means that most clinicians are without access to such sophisticated equipment. It should also be noted that the use of such instrumentation is not necessarily a completely objective measurement of the voice, as interpretation of data can be extremely subjective. Clinicians undertaking any sort of qualitative or perceptual analysis of a child's voice need to check their own observational and listening skills regularly to ensure reliability. This can be done informally with colleague(s) sharing a similar interest, thus preventing the problem of 'one man's moderate is another's severe'.

It cannot be stressed enough that it is essential to have a full and accurate diagnosis from an otolaryngologist prior to any intervention with the dysphonic child. A diagnosis of 'normal vocal folds' or 'no lesions seen' is not sufficient, and provides inadequate information about the actual functioning of the vocal folds and related structures. Ideally, children with dysphonia should be seen in a voice clinic with access to stroboscopy, an experienced speech & language therapist, and an interested otolaryngologist. This would not only enable the clinician to target the voice exercises more appropriately, but would also ensure the clinician does not spend weeks (or even months) working with the child with a cyst, for example, wondering why therapy was not effecting any change.

The purposes of a voice evaluation are as follows:

◆ To gain a detailed description of the child's voice characteristics, and how these characteristics vary over time.
◆ To determine the severity of the child's voice disorder.
◆ To determine whether or not the child would benefit from a programme of voice therapy
    (Adapted from Deem & Miller, 2000)

Voice Evaluation Process

The clinician working with dysphonic adults has a relatively easy task when it comes to assessment. The clinician can demonstrate certain tasks, and the client is usually able to imitate and cooperate. This may not be so easy to achieve with a child. The clinician therefore needs to spend time building up a relationship with the child prior to the assessment, just as when working with any child with a speech and/or language problem. It is essential to understand the parameters being assessed, as summarised in Table 2, and to design activities that will elicit the desired responses.

Table 2 Parameters for Assessment
Pitch range, optimal pitch and habitual pitch
Intensity (vocal loudness level)
Breath support and control
Rate of speech
Resonance
Sites of vocal tension/hyperfunction (supralaryngeal and laryngeal)
Quality of voice
Severity of dysphonia
Posture
Vocal stamina and flexibility
Articulatory features or problems

The authors have devised a 'quick and dirty' voice evaluation and assessment form (Appendix 2). Clinicians should be aware that this is a screening assessment form and that, unfortunately, there are no standardised tests available for clinicians to use during voice diagnosis. However, there are recognised 'gold standard' perceptual voice evaluation tools: the Vocal Profile Analysis (Laver et al, 1982), and the GRBAS (Hirano, 1981). We shall not attempt to describe each of the parameters to be assessed in any depth, as there are many other excellent texts that do so (Boone, 1980; Martin & Lockhart, 2000). We shall, however, note some of the relevant behaviours embedded in each of the parameters, and explain some ways in which these may be elicited.

Pitch and Range

Listen to the child's pitch in general conversation or while talking to their parent or guardian, or playing with a sibling. Ask the child to hum at a variety of different pitches, after being given an example. If higher pitched hums are clearer, it may be that the child has developed the use of a lower habitual pitch, which is putting some additional tension on the vocal folds. Try to coax the child to sing a short song, such as 'Happy Birthday', which even the youngest child will often be keen to do. Notice the pitch variability within the song, as a restricted pitch range is often a sign of vocal pathology. Perhaps try asking the child to go up and down a scale with you, using a ladder for going up and a snake for going down. Observe a smooth glide down, and note any pitch breaks.

Intensity (Vocal Loudness Levels)

Listening to the child playing is an excellent way to assess the parameter of vocal loudness, as most children will use a variety of different volumes even within one game! See if the child can vary the volume and use a quieter voice (as if they were in a library) without using a whisper. A child with tissue changes – such as nodules, polyps or oedema – may have great difficulty with softer sounds, since it is difficult for the vocal folds to approximate evenly without considerable effort. Also notice any hard glottal attacks, which are often present with this increase in effort.

Breath Support and Control

Observation of the child at rest will usually give the clinician an idea of the kind of breathing pattern the child is using. Do not be tempted to ask the child to take a 'deep breath', because this will often result in an immediate increase in shoulder tension, and clavicular breathing will occur. It can also result in what the authors call 'noisy hands-up'(the slight gasp with air intake that children usually make when putting their hands up excitedly in class); this noise on air intake is due to tense laryngeal musculature, as the vocal folds are not fully abducting on inspiration.

If the child is old enough, ask them to count up to three, then five, then 10, then 20, and look at the use of air and observe whether or not the child can control it or if replenishing breaths are taken. There is some debate about the usefulness of the s/z ratio, but it can be useful to look at the way the child supports phonation. This can be elicited, even with the younger child, by using a snake going into its cave for the 's', and a bee going into its hive for the 'z'.

When focusing on breathing, and in particular on how a child uses that air for voice, it is important to look at the rate of speech. A child who talks extremely fast will often not stop to take a 'top-up' breath, and tends to continue talking until they are speaking on residual air.

Resonance

In order for the clinician to gain an accurate description of the child's resonance, they may have to test specifically for hyper- and hyponasality. Ask the child to say sentences with no nasal sounds, such as 'Charlie has a fat cat.' Is there any difference with the nostrils occluded? Does the resonance sound appropriate? When looking at hyponasality, look to see whether or not the child is a mouth-breather. Ask them to say a sentence loaded with nasals – for example, 'my nose never runs'. Eliciting a hum will give the clinician an idea about the presence of any nasal obstruction, and is a useful way of seeing whether or not the child can actually increase the nasal resonance by feeling the vibrations around the nose. Listen to the child's ability to change their oral-nasal resonance during connected speech, and also note the overall balance of resonance.

Quality of Voice and Phonation

Sustained phonation using the vowel 'ah' will give the clinician information about the actual voice quality, and allow them to ascertain whether or not the child exhibits any voice breaks or diplophonia. Most young children can sustain a voiced sound such as 'z' for about 10 seconds (Andrews, 1986). Also listen to the onset of the note, and for the presence of any hard glottal onset, as discussed earlier. Or use a sentence such as 'Uncle Eddie eats eggs.' If a child appears to be using excessive effort during phonation, note any observable signs of tension in the jaw, neck or shoulders. Observe the vocal quality in connected speech, noting whether the voice is harsh, breathy or creaky, and if so to what degree (mild, moderate, severe).

Notice the quality and flexibility of the voice as the session continues, as this tells you about vocal stamina. It may also be worth seeing the child at different times of the day, to see whether their voice is better, for example, first thing in the morning.

Posture and Tension

Inappropriate muscle tension is often the result of poor posture. It is therefore essential that the clinician assesses the child's general body posture, as well as head and neck alignment. As mentioned in Chapter 2, poor posture may be more significant in children because of sedentary lifestyles: more time is spent sitting at a computer, watching the television, or playing on a playstation.

When assessing posture, look at the way the child sits, stands and moves; notice any increase in body tension as the child uses their voice, and observe the head position. An anterior head position with the chin tipped forward will directly affect the tension of the vocal folds. The child who talks with their head tipped to one side, or with their chin on their chest, may have reduced their resonating space. Observe any shoulder hunching or slouching, as this may create tension in the strap muscles and ultimately affect the voice.

Specific sites of tension that need to be observed include the jaw, tongue, pharynx and larynx, which are often (although not always) accompanied by general body tension. It is exceptionally difficult for the inexperienced clinician to 'home in' on the specific sites of tension, but most will pick up on the fact that the voice sounds 'tight', 'squeezed', or 'forced'. A useful tip when assessing any child with a voice disorder, is to try to mimic the voice that the child is producing. Ideally the clinician needs to have developed their own kinaesthetic feedback skills if this is going to be a useful tool. Work by Estill (1995) has contributed enormously to the understanding of the effect of individual muscle groups on the vocal apparatus, and enables clinicians to recognise and locate the degree of work involved in their own voice production.

Excessive muscle tension in and around the jaw will affect articulation and resonance. The placement of the tongue for speech is critical, as a retracted tongue position may occlude the pharynx and affect resonance. A more forward tongue position not only affects the resonance and quality of the back vowels, but also elevates the larynx, which will 'tighten up' the vocal folds.

A fairly accurate diagnostic symptom of tension within the laryngeal area is an 'ache' or 'discomfort', so it is important to ask the child if they are experiencing any pain when they use their voice, and if so where it 'hurts'. If the child presents with a strained or pressed vocal quality, or any hard glottal attack, this may be a sign of increased laryngeal tension.

The Voice Clinic

As mentioned earlier, ideally children should be assessed in a voice clinic with access to videostroboscopy. However, a recent survey presented by Rattenbury (2001) at the Newcastle Voice Therapy Conference found that only 9 per cent of speech and language therapy services had access to a voice clinic. Eighty-one per cent of voice referrals (adult and paediatric) were from general ENT clinics. So the reality is quite different from the ideal.

If the child has been referred to a voice clinic, and the clinician is able to see the child prior to the appointment, or even to go along with them, then the clinician has a role in preparing the child for the clinic. We do not intend to go into detail about voice clinics but clinicians may wish to refer to *The Voice Clinic Handbook* (Harris *et al*, 2000).

We have produced a 'Voice Clinic Information Leaflet' (Appendix 3), which is useful to give to parents or guardians prior to the appointment, and will help them explain to their child what will actually happen.

Chapter 4: Principles of Therapy and Management

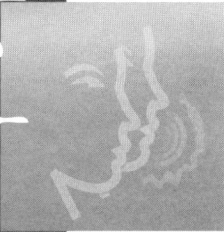

INTRODUCTION

Following the completion of a comprehensive assessment of the child and their dysphonia, the clinician now needs to use their skill and expertise in deciding on an appropriate course of action. Issues needing to be addressed include:

◆ Appropriateness of intervention

◆ Frequency of intervention

◆ Duration of treatment

◆ General aims of intervention

◆ Specific aims for the individual child

◆ Prognosis.

This chapter looks at the above areas to enable the clinician to make the necessary clinical decisions.

DECISION TO INTERVENE

The clinician's decision on whether or not to intervene is never straightforward, and requires the balancing of several, possibly contradictory, factors. As evidence-based practice develops, the clinician can turn to a range of documentation and studies. However, because childhood communication problems need to take account of the developmental aspect of a child's life, they cause most debate. The efficacy of treatment of vocal nodules in adults is well-documented (McCrory, 2001; Ramig & Verdolini, 1998), but the debate continues for childhood nodules. For example, should the tendency of nodules to disappear by the end of adolescence, particularly in boys, be an argument against surgical intervention (Pannbacker, 1999)? Von Leden (1985) stated that 'surgery has no place in the treatment of most vocal nodules occurring in children', and certainly the use of anaesthetics and a hospital stay should not be undertaken lightly. In addition, the continuation of poor vocal use by the child would indicate a likely return of the problem; this is supported by the authors' experience with the child outlined in Case Summary 5 (pp31–32). Sander (1989) argues against any type of intervention, suggesting that a trained listener detects hoarseness either not apparent to other listeners, or accepted by them as within normal limits. He theorises that any detectable hoarseness may be a result of normal developmental processes in the larynx. Kay (1982) questions the value of speech and language therapy intervention, deeming it to be 'insignificant', and concludes that neither therapy nor surgery has any more effect than leaving children alone.

In contrast to these views, Mori (1999) states that surgical intervention is the only reliable way to gain any improvement in voice quality prior to puberty, although post puberty there is no measurable difference in outcome between vocal hygiene advice, surgery and therapy only. Sarfati and Auday (1996) identified that nodules persist into adulthood for girls, by which time poor vocal behaviours are well entrenched, and also noted that puberty does not automatically resolve nodules in boys. Kahane and Mayo (1989) argue against the position taken by Sander (1989), and state categorically that speech and language therapy can eliminate vocal abuse and reduce existing lesions. Miller and Madison (1984) recorded a success rate of 75 per cent in eliminating nodules by therapy.

In 1987, Moran and Pentz surveyed otolaryngologists on the role of voice therapy in the treatment of nodules. Although there was a low response rate, there was an overwhelming preference for surgery for adults, but a preference was expressed for a wider range of choices for the treatment of children (Table 3).

Table 3 Options for the Treatment of Vocal Nodules	
Treatment Options	Percentage
Voice therapy alone	59
Surgery plus voice therapy	10
No direct intervention	15
Voice rest	2
Counselling by the physician	2
'Other'	12

Of the otolaryngologists, 63 per cent believed speech & language therapists were adequately trained to deliver voice therapy, but while 66 per cent always referred to them, 8 per cent advised against speech and language therapy.

Although Sander (1989) identifies a legitimate concern regarding the trained listener, it is too simplistic to assign all children's voice problems to a developmental process. There are degrees of hoarseness, and the child who suffers with periods of aphonia, and an unreliable voice for much of the time, should not be denied help. The authors believe that the effect of poor voice quality on the child is far reaching, touching as it does on the development of self-expression, personality, and the establishment and maintenance of social relationships. In both the social and educational aspects of their lives, children have as complex an existence as any adult. It is therefore vital that the child is able to participate fully in the development of all these aspects of their life. There appears to be a general consensus away from surgical intervention, and the authors have been fortunate to work alongside an otolaryngologist who strongly supports speech and language therapy. The therapy option is one that can produce effective outcomes for children, and is less distressing than surgery for child and family alike.

APPROACHES TO THERAPY

Individual therapy offers the opportunity for very specifically targeted tasks, whereas the group approach increases the options for more naturalistic communication settings, and thereby improves the chances for generalisation of skills. The nature of voice therapy with children is comparable to one style of working with dysfluent children. Both approaches aim to change the manner in which the child communicates. Neither produces instant results, and both present the clinician with huge challenges in maintaining motivation during therapy as well as improvements following therapy. The authors believe that the group setting offers many benefits:

◆ The motivation of the children is improved by the element of peer support, since few children have met others with similar problems.

◆ There are opportunities for a wider range of activities that are more fun for the children.

◆ There is the ability to set up 'mock' communication settings, such as talking in a classroom, to practise newly acquired skills.

◆ Information is presented in a more manageable way for the children, as there is not the intensity of the one-to-one therapy situation.

◆ The setting is less intimidating for the children than an adult-child interaction.

Therapy is, however, the art of applying knowledge to varying individuals, settings, circumstances and needs. For some children and their families the group situation is not the best option – for example, if the children needing therapy do not form a cohesive group, or if there are particular circumstances preventing attendance at a group. Alternatively, some children may not respond well in the group setting, and individual sessions would result in a better outcome, as demonstrated in Case Summary 3 (p24). The clinician should be able to adapt the strategies and ideas from the group setting for the individual session.

The child's parent or main carer should be present and involved in the discussions on the way the voice works. Decisions on incorporating changes in vocal use into everyday life should be made by the parent or carer and the child, with the clinician taking the role of a facilitator, keeping targets realistic and achievable.

The entire voice care programme, which will be discussed in greater depth in later chapters, must be broken down into its components. No more than one or two of these should be tackled at a time by the child and family. In this way the programme will be completed in manageable stages.

PRINCIPLES OF THERAPY

The therapeutic approaches that work with adults are also appropriate for use with children – that is to say, there is no mystery to improving a child's voice. All that the clinician needs to know is how to communicate the necessary ideas and information in a way appropriate for each child. The principles of voice therapy with children may be summarised as follows:

◆ To make complex, abstract ideas used in adult therapy more concrete and therefore more understandable for children.

◆ To enable the practice of new skills in as natural a way as possible.

◆ To make the changes in vocal behaviour relevant to the child and their family.

Therapy should aim to enable the child and their family to make any adjustments or changes to vocal behaviour that might be necessary for the improvement of voice quality as simply and effectively as possible. Expertise in voice therapy tends to develop among clinicians working with adult case-loads, and it can be difficult to adjust to working with children with voice disorders. Most adults respond well to information about their voice and how it works, and some technical or 'jargon' words may actually be helpful. However, when working with children, some of the information presented to them in the most effective manner may appear, to the purist, to be inaccurate. It is imperative to remember that the message is of overriding importance. The slight inaccuracy of a few descriptions of anatomy, or physiological processes, is of little relevance when compared with enabling a child to grasp the theory of voice production and the principles of vocal hygiene.

THERAPY AIMS

The key to any successful therapy is to set realistic goals which are achievable and relevant to the individual receiving the therapy. Successful therapy outcomes are more likely to be maintained when an individual is well motivated and has the necessary self-esteem. The authors use *WHO-Enderby Therapy Outcome Measures* (Enderby, 1997, see form in Appendix 4), for which a typical long-term aim would be:

Voice quality acceptable to child and family.

Again, as with dysfluent children, fundamental changes in communication behaviour will be required, which in turn need a certain level of understanding and insight to succeed. There is also a considerable involvement of home and social factors. These may mean that clinicians need to allow themselves to succeed in a small goal if the larger goal is unrealistic. For example, the clinician may be able to instil the necessary theory for preventing vocal abuse and misuse, but the child is unable or unwilling to make use of it. It is acceptable to have as short-term therapy goals:

To be of aware of how the voice works
To be aware of what is 'good' and 'bad' for the voice.

Achieving these goals can improve the child's voice to a point at which it is acceptable to both the child and their parent or guardian, although the clinician may still feel that there is room for improvement. At this point the clinician should remember Sander (1989), and be aware that the presenting voice problem may not be as significant to untrained listeners. As in all therapy, the aim is not to achieve perfection, and the clinician may have to be content with preventing further deterioration in voice quality, and in beginning to adapt maladaptive vocal behaviour.

IMPLEMENTATION OF THERAPY

Once the decision to intervene has been made and appropriate goals set, the clinician has to decide the way in which therapy is delivered. The approach to voice therapy is predicated on three main factors (Pannbacker, 1998):

◆ Diagnosis

◆ Characteristics of the client (and, for children, the family)

◆ Preferred option of the clinician, including any bias towards a particular therapeutic approach.

However, it may be helpful to offer some guidance on implementing therapy.

Duration of Therapy Sessions

In each therapy session the clinician should present a new idea with sufficient explanation and opportunity to practise any exercises. Some areas are interrelated, and it therefore makes sense to cover more than one topic at a time – for example, posture and breathing. Other subjects are linked by opposition and make more sense when covered together – for example, tension and relaxation. When making these decisions, the clinician must always keep in mind the complexity of the information being delivered. It is far better to cover a small, discrete topic well, and ensure that it is fully understood, than to cover a wide range of information several times.

1 For children under seven years of age, when seen individually, 20–30 minutes is long enough for them to concentrate and take in all the new information.

2 Beyond seven years of age, the length of time can extend to around 45 minutes. Any more than this is usually not helpful.

3 In a group setting, children as young as four years of age can manage 1.5 hours, and in this format more information can be imparted. There is also greater scope for practising new techniques or suggestions.

Frequency of Therapy Sessions

It is generally acknowledged that intensive therapy in groups is the preferred option. While once a week for four weeks is not strictly speaking 'intensive', children are able to achieve a considerable amount. If this is followed by a consolidation break of 4–6 weeks, this allows the child and family the opportunity to try to maintain vocal improvements gained in the group, and become at ease with implementing the vocal hygiene programme as part of everyday life.

However, individual sessions – because of the need to impart information in more manageable and smaller 'chunks' – necessitate longer practice times in order to incorporate the hygiene programme into everyday life. It may be that the clinician sees the child every two weeks, or even once a month, thereby ensuring that each part of the programme is fully understood and implemented before moving on.

The therapy delivered to children in groups, or individually, is centred on a voice modification programme (Appendix 5). The main features of this programme are:

- Avoid shouting
- Use good posture and breathing
- Avoid whispering
- Ensure voice rest
- Avoid coughing or throat clearing
- Avoid hard onset.

A star chart (Appendix 6), which employs visual, positive reinforcement supports the implementation of this programme.

The following chapters will address the implementation of the star chart, and suggest various activities to establish and maintain the vocal hygiene programme.

Chapter 5: Developing a Programme of Vocal Hygiene for Children

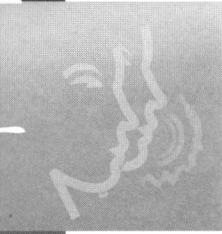

INTRODUCTION

The activities in the following three chapters are designed to:

◆ Establish an understanding of how the voice is produced

◆ Identify vocally abusive behaviour

◆ Enable the child to begin to modify elements of misuse.

The activities are grouped under specific tasks, which support each aim and include suggested vocabulary to use. By following this programme, supported by the star chart (Appendix 6), trauma to the vocal apparatus should be reduced and vocal nodules eliminated.

The authors believe that an understanding of the anatomy of voice and how to modify vocal behaviour, including voice rest, provide the essential foundations for any further exercises.

ANATOMY

The first step is to establish an understanding of the way in which the voice is produced, before concentrating on the way in which the child is producing their voice.

Vocabulary: making voice

voice box

muscles

lungs.

ACTIVITIES TO ESTABLISH STRUCTURES
USED IN VOICE PRODUCTION

1   Copy and cut out the body outline and the shapes of the voice box and the
    lungs (Appendix 8). Ask the child to put the shapes on the body where they
    think they belong. In the group, explain that the voice box is in the neck, or
    throat; that air is drawn in and out of the lungs as we breathe, and that the
    sound of the voice is made as air comes out of the lungs, over the voice box.

2   Ask the child to point to their own voice box and lungs.

3   Ask the child to draw a person, and show where the parts are that make the
    voice. Can the child name these parts?

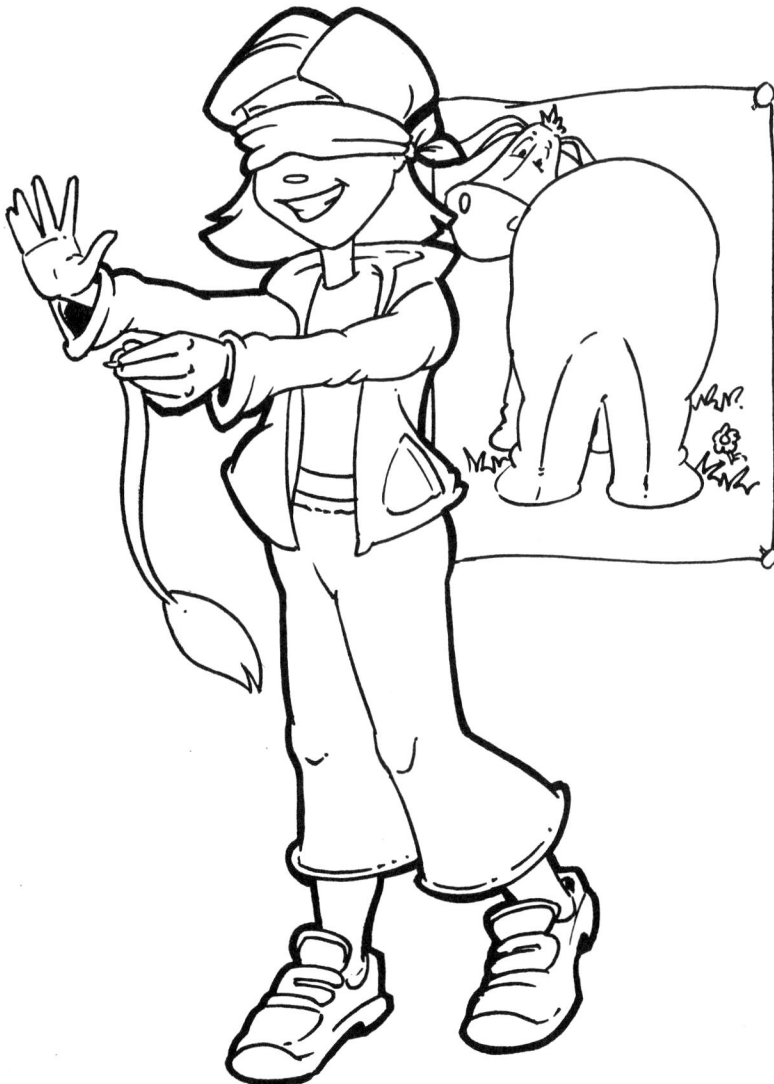

ACTIVITIES TO ESTABLISH AN UNDERSTANDING OF THE WAY THAT THE LUNGS WORK

1   Blow up a balloon to demonstrate how the lungs expand when air is drawn in. Draw the child's attention to the rise and fall of their own chest as they breathe. Use a piece of string or a tape measure to see how much the balloon grows.

2   Repeat the exercise, this time putting the balloon inside a plastic bag. Ensure the bag is smaller than the expanded balloon (the sort used at serve-yourself vegetable or sweet counters are suitable). Measure the size of the balloon when it is blown up inside the bag. Draw the child's attention to the way the amount of air in the balloon is reduced by the constriction of the bag.

3   Use the body outline and lung cut-outs to draw attention to the shape of the lungs. Which part of the lungs can hold the most air? Where is this on the child's own body?

ACTIVITIES TO ESTABLISH AN UNDERSTANDING OF WHAT MAKES THE VOICE BOX AND LUNGS WORK

1   The child needs to understand what a muscle is. The aim is for them to understand that a muscle causes movement. Ask the child to make various movements, for example:

◆ Smile

◆ Raise a hand

◆ Stick tongue in and out

◆ Walk

◆ Shrug shoulders.

Explain that muscles also make the lungs draw air in and out, and help the voice box make a voice as the air passes through it.

Older children should be able to cope with an explanation of the vocal folds and how they work, and if the child understands that they have nodules on their vocal folds then it is worth describing this to them. However, this can confuse younger children, and it is enough to say that air passes through the voice box to make sound.

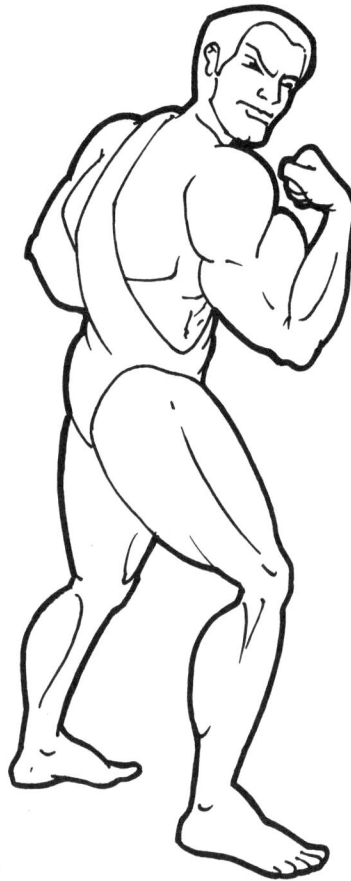

2   Stretch out two pieces of elastic, side by side, for the children to 'twang'. Repeat with thread, thin string, or twine. Compare these to the vocal folds, and explain that muscles 'hold' the ends of the elastic and the air 'twangs' the vocal folds.

VOICE REST

The rationale for voice rest in adults is debatable, as it is effective only while being implemented, unless used in conjunction with therapy to change patterns of muscle misuse (Mathieson, 2001). However, voice rest in children has different aims:

◆ To establish the voice as something over which the child has control, that is, by choosing not to use it.

◆ To encourage the child to take responsibility for looking after their voice. For example, by resting it if they detect a deterioration in voice quality.

Vocabulary: tired muscles

tense muscles

relaxed muscles.

ACTIVITIES TO ESTABLISH WHAT VOICE REST IS AND HOW TO DO IT

1 Ask the child to try to make as many different kinds of sound as possible. For example, talk, hum, sing, laugh, cry, sounds of surprise (aha). Point out that *all* sounds from the mouth are made by the voice box, not just talking.

2 Ask the child to do the following activities: stand on one leg for a short time; clench fists; walk round and round the room, and put their hand in the air. Discuss whether they could do such activities all afternoon or all day. Explain that this would be hard to do because their muscles would get very tired. In the same way, the muscles working the voice box and lungs get tired talking, and need to rest. The therapist should stress that lungs get tired pushing air out for talking, *not* for ordinary breathing.

3 Set up a quiet activity such as puzzles, or drawing a picture, to demonstrate to the child what is meant by complete voice rest. Discuss with the child and parent or carer a realistic target for daily voice rest. The most important aim is to establish a daily routine, although it is often better to propose voice rest on weekdays only as most families find it can be more difficult to keep to a routine at the weekend. Suggested targets could be from two minutes per day up to about 10 minutes per day.

4 Brainstorm ideas on how to gain attention when resting the voice. For example, by clapping hands, or moving nearer to the person that they are talking to.

5 Brainstorm ideas on how to ask for something when resting the voice. For example, through gesture or mime.

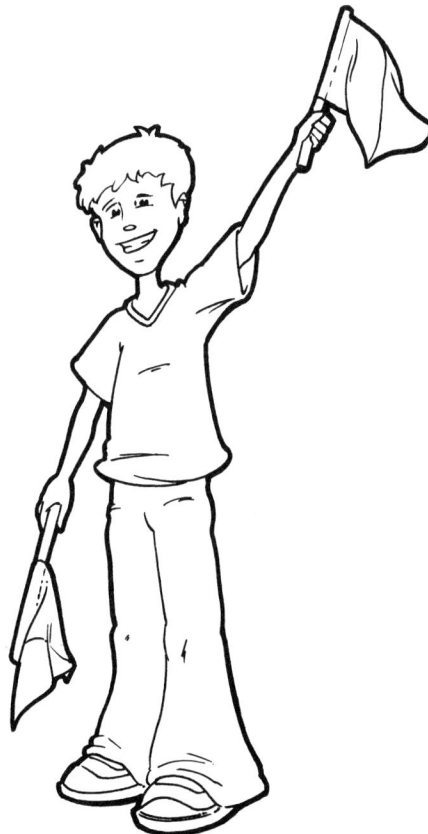

MODIFYING VOCAL ABUSE AND MISUSE

The aim of this part of the programme is to help the child to establish an appropriate volume; however, there will always be circumstances when shouting is unavoidable. The child needs to be given an alternative such as a 'calling' voice – that is, use of a 'sing-song' or intoned voice. This is less stressful on the voice, and at the same time enables the child to be heard. Clinicians who have been appropriately trained may wish to use 'Yellwell' pioneered by Alison Bagnell (1982).

Vocabulary: quiet voice

gentle voice

loud voice

whisper

hammering voice

cough or throat clear.

ACTIVITIES TO ESTABLISH AUDITORY DISCRIMINATION AND SELF-MONITORING SKILLS

1   Use a ColorCards® *Listening Skills* set (*Indoor* or *Outdoor Sounds*) or similar, matching sounds to pictures, or a tape made within the department. Begin with activity of gross discrimination – of, for example, a telephone ringing, a person whistling, crumpling paper, or a banging door – and ask the child to decide whether a noise is loud or quiet. This activity can also be incorporated into practice of voice rest by using gesture to indicate the choice. The child can develop their own gestures – for example, hands over ears for loud, and the thumbs up sign for a quiet or gentle voice.

2   Make a tape of sentences read out in a mixture of loud voices, quiet voices, hammering voices (hard glottal attack), and whispers. Clinicians who feel more comfortable talking about hard attack should be aware that a visual mime of 'hammering' helps the child to appreciate it more quickly. The clinician should demonstrate this before beginning the tape. Again, encourage the use of gesture – for example, a whisper could be a finger held vertically across the lips; a hammering mime could indicate a hard attack.

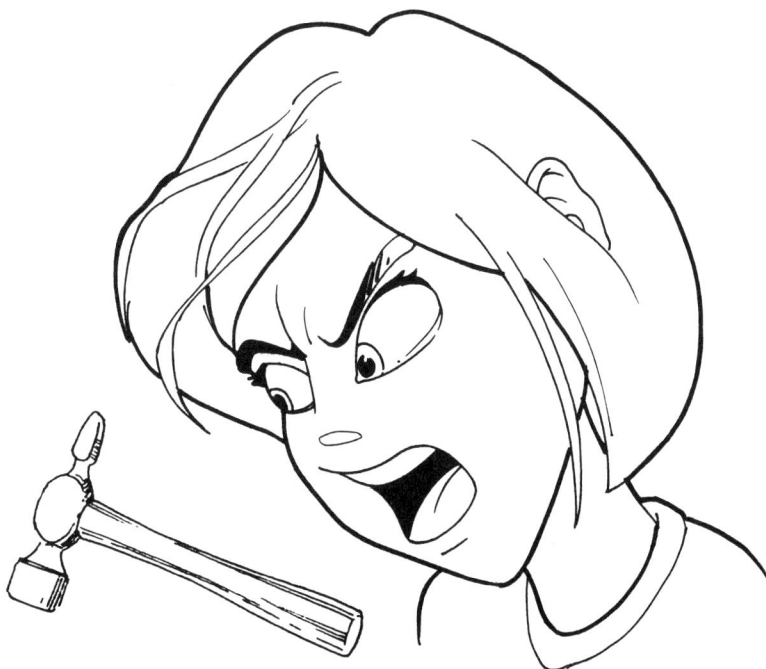

ACTIVITIES TO ESTABLISH AUDITORY DISCRIMINATION AND SELF-MONITORING SKILLS *(continued)*

3 Make a tape of single words read out in a loud voice, a quiet voice, a hammering voice, or a whisper. Can the child still discriminate reliably?

4 Use enlarged pictures from the star chart (Appendix 7), and place them around the room. When the clinician says a sentence or a single word, the child moves to the appropriate picture. Whenever a verbal activity takes place, the child is to be encouraged to decide what kind of voice has been used, by others as well as themselves.

5 Using large verb pictures (such as the Colorcards® *Verbs* series), ask each child to take one, and to mime the verb on the card for the rest of the group to guess.

6 Ask each child to think of a simple sentence – for example, 'The water is blue.' Ask them to say it using an angry voice, perhaps as if the water *should* be red, and then to say the same sentence using a gentle voice, as if blue is their favourite colour. Discuss what they can 'feel' physically, and aim to draw out the differences in tension, volume and so on.

7 Practise using a gentle voice in any number of verbal games, for example:
   ◆ I went on holiday and I packed ...
   ◆ The doctor's cat is a ... cat
   ◆ I went to the shops and I bought ...
   ◆ Twenty questions.

Encourage the children to rate the type of voice used by themselves, and each other.

8 Use sequencing cards (eg, ColorCards®), and ask each child to tell the story to the rest of the group. Encourage the children to rate each other's voice, as

ACTIVITIES TO ESTABLISH AUDITORY DISCRIMINATION AND SELF-MONITORING SKILLS *(continued)*

well as their own.

9 Describe to the child what is meant by throat-clearing or coughing, and establish the difference between a persistent habit and the necessity of coughing with a cold. Discuss and, as necessary, practise alternatives, such as a sip of water, a hard swallow, or a silent throat clear.

10 Having established what hard glottal attack is, discuss how using a lower volume can reduce this. Incorporate this practice into the voice exercises. Other techniques include:

◆ Producing consonant–vowel (CV) structures, using *h* plus vowel. This allows the child to begin the airflow during the voiceless phoneme and add voice gradually. Ensure that the CV structure does not become too breathy. Use open, relaxed vowels – avoiding, for example, *ee*, as these are particularly susceptible to hard attack when they occur in the initial position of a stressed syllable.

◆ Using breathy onset of words, for example $s \rightarrow z$, $f \rightarrow v$, or $h \rightarrow m$.

◆ Eventually practise reducing hard attack in sentences such as:

Ian the ostrich eats ivy.

Uncle Arthur acts appallingly.

Ivor the Engine eagerly waits.

Alyson and Edward ate the apples.

I open eggs at Easter.

Annie ape always argues.

Auntie Anne is ugly.

Elephants always eat ants.

Is Eddie always angry?

Eskimos' igloos are icy.

SUMMARY

Vocal hygiene is the pivotal point of intervention for childhood dysphonia. The success of further therapy, as outlined in Chapters 6–8, depends upon the successful implementation of the ideas contained in this chapter. If a programme of vocal hygiene is not initiated and established, then any further therapy will not be effective and will result in a poor therapy outcome.

Chapter 6: Relaxation and Posture Modification

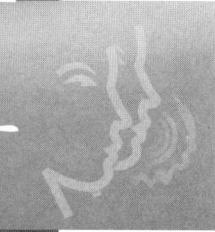

INTRODUCTION

Chapters 6, 7 and 8 focus on strategies to enhance relaxation and improve breath control for voice, and voice therapy techniques. However, it is important to remember that although a programme of vocal hygiene underpins any voice work, Chapters 6, 7 and 8 should not be viewed as a recipe book. The intention is for the clinician to use the exercises suggested selectively, according to the presentation of the dysphonia.

AIMS OF THERAPY

For the majority of children, the way in which they sit, stand or move has little relevance, as the days of walking with a book on the head to improve posture are long gone. However, for the child with a voice problem, posture is of great importance, because inappropriate muscular tension is frequently generated by poor posture.

The aim of the clinician is to help the child become aware of any tension within their body, and to enable the child to reduce this tension. Most children, on being told to stand up straight, adopt a rigid posture with chest pushed out and shoulders raised. The clinician must relate any work done on posture and relaxation to the production of voice, as explained in the preceding chapter. That is, the muscles used in producing voice need to be appropriately balanced (relaxed) and used in the best possible way.

Working on posture and relaxation also enables children to develop their proprioceptive skills, which are particularly useful when moving on to work on specific voice therapy techniques (see Chapter 8). The ability to self-monitor will not only help the child to self-correct poor posture, but also to decrease muscular tension.

POSTURE

Vocabulary: tense

relaxed or floppy

low shoulders

straight lungs or crumpled lungs

heavy arms or legs.

ACTIVITIES TO ESTABLISH AN AWARENESS
OF TENSION IN THE BODY

1   Ask children to stand to attention like a soldier, and to keep still for two
    to three minutes. Then discuss what it felt like in their shoulders, back
    and limbs.

2   Ask children to imagine that
    they are a puppet, and that
    the strings attached to their
    arms have been cut.
    Discuss how heavy their
    arms felt, and how floppy
    they were.

3   Explain the contrast
    between tension and
    relaxation through the
    examples of cooked and
    uncooked spaghetti, an oak
    tree and a falling leaf, a
    statue and a lump of clay.

4   Using the activity of blowing up the balloon, discuss how the lungs can be
    prevented from working efficiently if they are not 'straight' – that is, if they are
    'crumpled up'.

5   Play a shrugging game, in which one child volunteers to be the 'spotter'. Hand
    out a piece of paper or card to each of the other children, one of which is
    marked with ↑. The 'spotter' turns away, and the child with the marked card
    slightly raises one or both shoulders and holds the position. The 'spotter' then
    has to decide who has shrugged, and whether with one or both shoulders.
    This game raises an awareness of shoulder position and how to alter it.

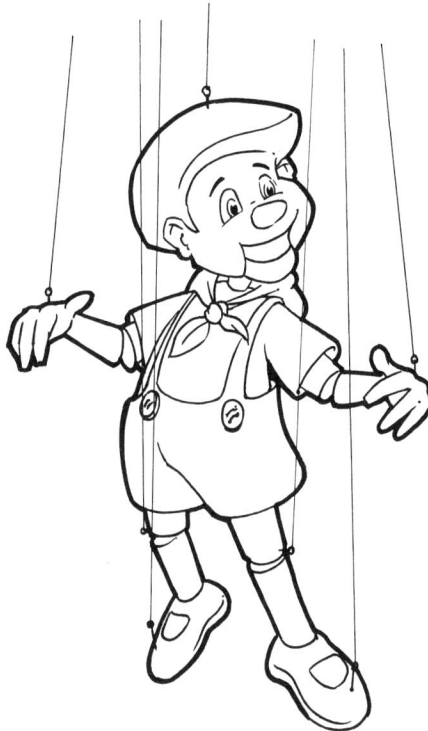

ACTIVITIES TO ESTABLISH AN AWARENESS OF TENSION IN THE BODY *(continued)*

6 Ask each child to find a new way of sitting on a chair. Ask them how comfortable it is, particularly if they hold the position for a few minutes.

7 Ask the children to find a comfortable position sitting on the chair that gives them straight lungs. Explain that they will always be asked to sit like this in the therapy sessions.

8 Play a game of 'Going to...'. Each child takes it in turns to move around the room as if they were going:

◆ To a party

◆ To a circus

◆ To lay the table for tea

◆ To tidy their room

◆ To be late for school

◆ To walk on the beach

◆ To get the last ice-cream.

The rest of the group has to decide whether the child is tense or relaxed, and why. The clinician should try to draw out that tension could also result from being excited.

ACTIVITIES TO ESTABLISH AN AWARENESS OF TENSION IN THE BODY (continued)

9 Discuss how twisting the neck or holding the head at a funny angle can stop the voice 'muscles' from working properly. Allow the child to try talking with their chin tucked well down, and with their head stretched up like a giraffe.

10 Stand the child with their back and shoulders against a wall, and then help them to allow the head to come forward about two centimetres. Encourage the child to try to find this neutral head position for the larynx, themselves.

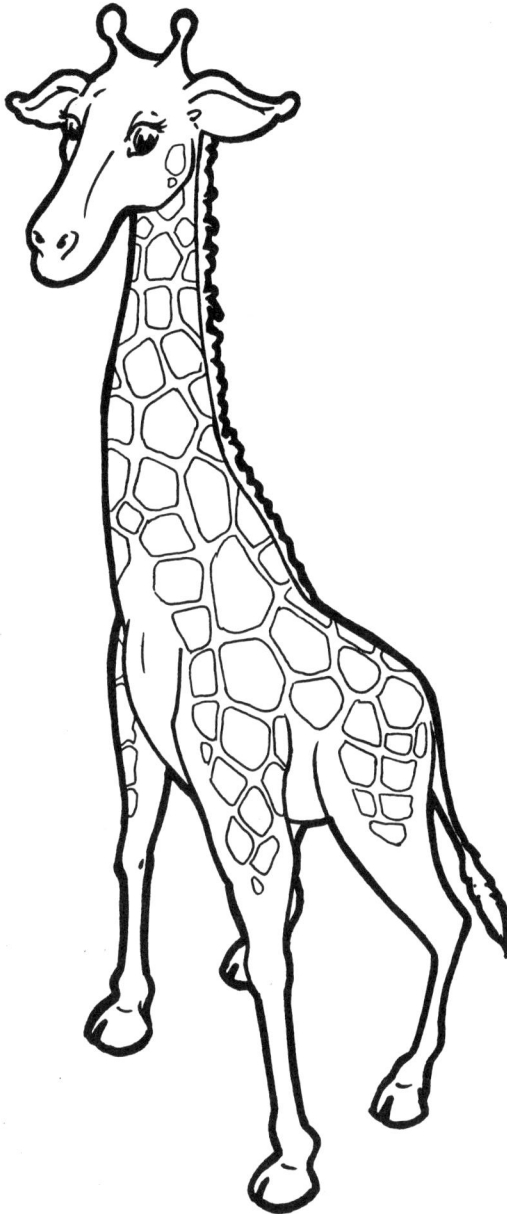

RELAXATION

Vocabulary: tense

relaxed or floppy

low shoulders

heavy arms or legs

slowly and gently.

ACTIVITIES TO ENCOURAGE THE CHILD'S AWARENESS OF TENSION AND HOW IT RELATES TO BODY POSITION, AND TO INTRODUCE RELAXATION

1   Begin by using facial grimaces to identify tension in facial muscles.

2   Have the child imagine a pencil is attached to the end of each shoulder in turn, and ask them to roll their shoulder *gently*, to draw imaginary circles in the air.

3   Have the child gently draw one shoulder up to touch their ear, and hold for a few seconds, before relaxing it down slowly and gently. Repeat with the other shoulder.

4   If mats or rugs are available, it is possible to attempt full body relaxation. Turn off the lights and close any blinds or curtains. When the child is lying down, the clinician can, using a slow calm voice, talk the child through full body relaxation. Explain to the children that a clinician may move around the room to check, or help them, with arm and leg relaxation.

Clinicians may wish to use the following script:

◆   Slowly and gently screw up your face and hold it (for a few seconds). Now gently relax.

◆   Gently raise your shoulders up to your ears; hold them, and now relax.

◆   Gently pull in your tummy button. Can you feel the middle of your back against the floor? Now, slowly let it come back up.

◆   Clench your hands into fists; hold them tightly, and slowly uncurl your fingers and relax your hands.

◆   Stretch your toes down towards the floor, and gently relax.

◆   Now pull up your toes towards your chin; hold them there, and now let your feet flop.

ACTIVITIES TO ENCOURAGE THE CHILD'S AWARENESS OF TENSION AND HOW IT RELATES TO BODY POSITION, AND TO INTRODUCE RELAXATION *(continued)*

This will work better if the children keep their eyes closed and try to keep the parts of the body still once they have been dealt with.

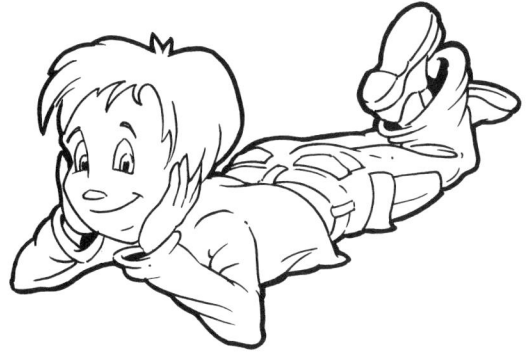

5   Once a child is fully relaxed, it is worth trying some imagery. Children can respond very well to images that are appropriate to them. The clinician needs to describe the image in great detail, using a slow and calm voice, and painting a verbal picture for the child to visualise.

Images that have worked well include:

◆   Floating in a hot air balloon; talking about the feel of the sun, the sound of the breeze. Ask the child to imagine that they are watching a red car on a small twisty lane, going round bends, disappearing under trees for a few seconds. Describe how the trees look, the shiny, winding river, the cows in the field.

◆   Lying on an inflatable in a swimming pool on holiday. Describe the warmth of the sun, the gentle movement of the water, the far off sounds of children laughing in the sea, perhaps the sound of seabirds and the feeling of having nothing to do but float.

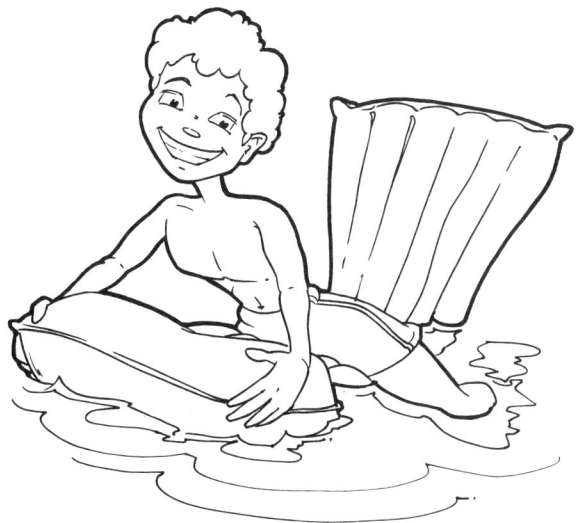

ACTIVITIES TO ENCOURAGE THE CHILD'S AWARENESS OF TENSION AND HOW IT RELATES TO BODY POSITION, AND TO INTRODUCE RELAXATION (continued)

◆ Lying in bed on the first day of the Winter holidays. Describe how cosy the bed feels; how soft the pillow is, and how the wind and rain sound outside the window. Talk about how good it feels to know that you can stay in bed and not get up for school, and imagine what will happen over the next few days.

Some children, particularly those who are older, can suggest their own images for the clinician to expand upon. Once the image is constructed, the clinician can leave the child, for a few moments, to maintain it for themselves.

It is vital that a child is brought out of this kind of imaging carefully and gently. For example, the hot air balloon can gradually drift down to earth, as they watch things appear larger and larger and hear more things such as car engines, birds singing and cows mooing, before landing with a gentle bump. Others can be drawn out by hearing Mum calling them to get up, come for lunch etc, with Mum gradually getting louder and closer, and more insistent. The child is then asked to open their eyes without getting up; then to sit up when they feel ready, and finally to get up off the floor.

SUMMARY

All of the above techniques are designed to induce more general, or global, physical and mental relaxation. It is worth mentioning here that in some cases, where the child presents with very specific areas of head, neck or vocal tract tension, palpation and manipulation of the musculature may be beneficial. This, however, should only be used by clinicians with considerable experience of these techniques and who have had appropriate training. It is also imperative that any 'hands on' work with children needs to be discussed with the parents, and appropriate explanations given to the child.

Throughout all relaxation exercises, the clinician must ensure that the child maintains slow, gentle movements and that they do not do anything that causes them any degree of pain or discomfort. Occasionally a child will try so hard that even gentle exercises become more of a strenuous workout.

Chapter 7: Breathing for Voice

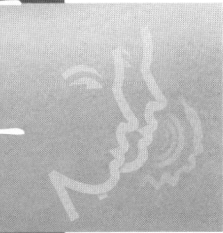

INTRODUCTION

In Chapter 1, we referred to the importance of breathing for voice and, although there is some controversy concerning 'breathing exercises' in voice therapy (Mathieson, 2001), children can benefit from these activities.

When working on children's breath support, the clinician should be aware of the child with asthma. For these children, drawing too much attention to breathing could trigger an attack, so although it is worth attempting these exercises, at the least sign of concern the activity should be stopped.

In our experience, it is unrealistic to attempt to achieve diaphragmatic breathing with children. Although some individuals may achieve it, the time needed to do this is better spent on other tasks. There is also the problem of a child, eager to please, actively pushing out their abdomen when breathing.

AIMS OF THERAPY

The aim of therapy is to improve the child's breath support and the control of airflow, and to practise the coordination of breathing and voicing. Before doing any breath activity, ensure that the child has a good posture, and be aware of the raising of shoulders and expanding of the upper chest as the child draws in a breath. It may be helpful to stand behind the child with hands resting on their shoulders, so that there is a tactile feedback if the shoulders start to rise. Standing next to the child, in front of a mirror, also enables the child to monitor their upper chest movement and compare it to that of the clinician.

Alternatively, lie the child flat on the floor to facilitate a lowered, relaxed carriage of the shoulders, and to decrease the likelihood of movement in the upper chest during inhalation.

ACTIVITIES TO INCREASE THE VOLUME OF AIR AVAILABLE FOR VOICING

1 Ask the child to imagine they are blowing a feather across the room on a continuous airstream. Time each child, to see who can blow the 'feather' the longest.

2 Ask the child to blow out a long line of candles, in one breath. This could be an imaginary line of candles, in view of safety considerations with real candles.

3 Use water-based paints and straws to blow patterns on paper.

4 If the use of candles is permitted, ask each child to blow a candle, not to extinguish the flame, but to make the flame 'dance'. This can also be turned into a competition as to whose candle dances longest.

5 Blow bubbles, and hold a competition to find out who can blow the biggest bubble before it bursts.

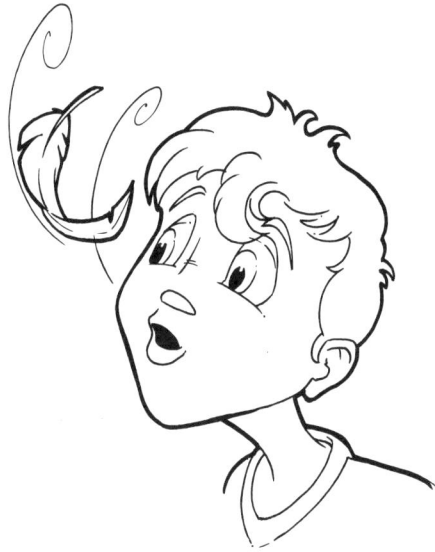

ACTIVITIES TO IMPROVE AIRSTREAM CONTROL

1 Ask the child to blow out a line of candles, with a different breath for each candle.

2 Use straws and small pieces of tissue paper to have a mini 'Blow Football Tournament' on a tabletop.

3 Use a line of candles, and ask the child to blow out alternate flames.

4 Use building blocks or small toys to create an obstacle course on the tabletop. Each child takes it in turns to blow a tissue 'ball' around the course, using a straw. Have a league table of the fastest time for completion of the course.

5 Stand the children in pairs, opposite each other. One child holds up a hand, palm facing their partner, with fingers spread. Their partner has to choose a finger, and blow air on to that finger alone.

Exercises using breath to write or draw in the air have been tried, but often result in much twisting and turning of the neck, and so are better not used.

ACTIVITIES TO ESTABLISH COORDINATION OF BREATH AND VOICING

1 The coordination of breath and voice requires control over the initiation of phonation. Begin by asking the child to move from a voiceless sound to a voiced sound, that is: $f \rightarrow v$, or $s \rightarrow z$. The voiceless fricative can then be removed. Decreased glottal resistance now results in a stronger airflow over the vocal folds. Other exercises can develop this skill further, for example:

Revving up a motorbike = *vvvvVVVV* (gradually increasing the volume of the 'revs')

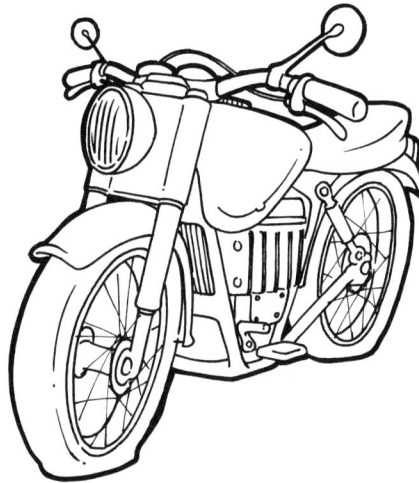

A bee flies towards you and then away = *zzzzZZZZzzzz*

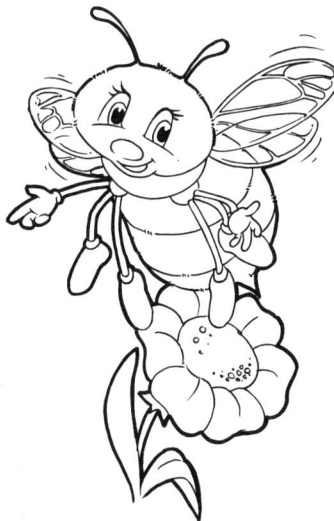

ACTIVITIES TO ESTABLISH COORDINATION OF BREATH AND VOICING *(continued)*

2 Begin by asking the child to produce *ah*. This activity can be extended into a competition by timing which child can maintain the vowel while keeping a good voice.

3 Demonstrate and practise using 'top-up' breaths. This will prevent laryngeal strain as the sub-glottic pressure begins to fail. For example: 1, 2, 3, 4 (top-up), 5, 6, 7, 8 (top-up), etc.

Ensure that the child does not gasp in air noisily, but uses a quick and quiet inhalation. This can be described to the child as the intake of breath that happens with a lovely surprise rather than a horrible shock.

Next try: 1, 2, 3 (top-up)

1, 2, 3, 4 (top-up)

1, 2, 3, 4, 5 (top-up)

1, 2, 3, 4, 5, 6 (top-up)

4 Using these breathing techniques, play verbal consequences. One child begins by making up a sentence; the next child adds a sentence, and so on round the group to make a story.

5 If you have a book of rhymes or limericks in the clinic, these are an excellent way to practise breathing for voice. Good books to have include Roald Dahl's *Revolting Rhymes* (2001), or any of Spike Milligan's children's verses (1973).

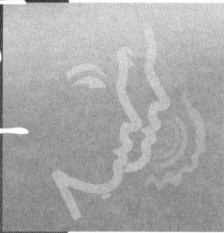

INTRODUCTION

In this chapter we focus on a variety of voice therapy techniques that can be used to correct specific patterns of laryngeal muscle misuse. Although most of these techniques have been tried and tested with dysphonic adults, the available literature makes little mention of the use of such techniques with children.

The choice of therapy technique, whether for an adult or a child, needs to be specific to the vocal pathology and the presenting pattern of muscle misuse. It is the authors' experience that many clinicians shy away from direct voice therapy techniques when working with the dysphonic child, preferring to focus more on indirect methods, such as those discussed in Chapter 5.

Traditionally, voice therapy tended to follow a prescriptive approach of relaxation, posture modification, breathing exercises, voice exercises and, finally, resonance and pitch work. However, more recent work completed by Harris *et al* (2000) has led to an increased understanding of the laryngeal mechanisms in normal function and dysfunction, enabling clinicians to direct their therapy more specifically.

It is our opinion that voice therapy with children need not always follow a prescriptive approach, and although the previous chapters cover the foundations for voice – for example, breath support and control, it is not always essential to go through these with every child as if working from a recipe book. If, for example, the child presents with an adequate posture and good breath control for phonation, the clinician can fairly swiftly move on to a more direct approach aimed at modifying the presenting muscle imbalance. However, in doing so, the clinician must continue to monitor the child closely, to ensure that while carrying out these exercises, they do not develop maladaptive behaviours, such as increased neck and shoulder tension.

The following techniques can be used when working with children individually, as well as in a group setting. In the latter, it is imperative that while the children carry out the exercises, the clinician observes them and modifies their technique accordingly. Ideally, we feel that two clinicians should run groups together, so that individual monitoring can be achieved, particularly when working on the actual voice production phase.

This chapter contains only a few of the voice therapy techniques available for clinicians to chose from, and is by no means complete. Those discussed are the ones that the authors prefer to use when working with dysphonic children, as they can be easily adapted. The chapter also covers some therapy ideas for working on resonance, pitch, vocal flexibility, and stamina.

ALTERING LARYNGEAL MUSCLE MISUSE

Humming/uh huh

Humming encourages the vocal tract to relax, in particular the areas above the level of the vocal folds. It is a good technique to encourage easy initiation of voice as the back of the vocal folds close gently together. It also helps to re-balance resonance by providing the child with some feelings of vibration in the mouth and nose, therefore taking the emphasis away from the larynx.

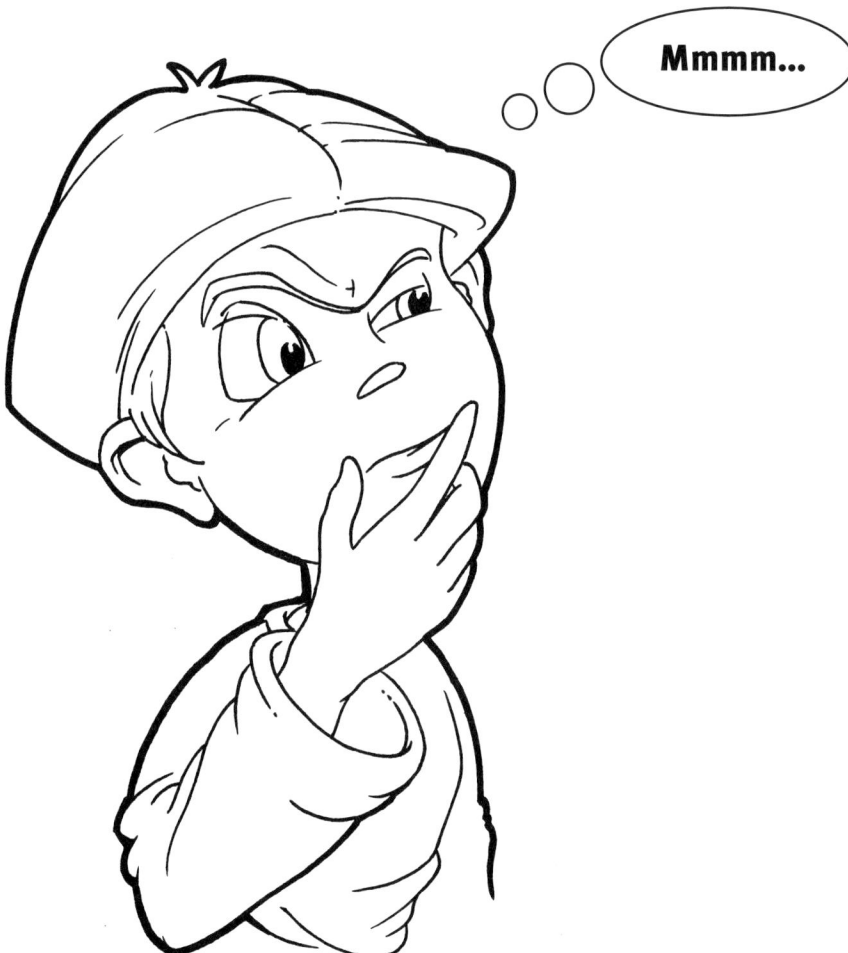

EXERCISES TO ESTABLISH THE HUMMING TECHNIQUE

1   It is often best to start this technique by encouraging children to use a soft onset prior to the initiation of the 'hum', to prevent a hard glottal onset. This can be done by asking the child to begin breathing down the nose and then add the hum.

2   Once this has been achieved, the hum can be prolonged (*mmm ...*), remembering that the lips should make light contact while the teeth remain apart. Encourage the child to imagine the sound forward on to their lips. This will allow the tongue to assume a neutral position, and because the hum is very close to quiet breathing, will also put the larynx in a neutral position.

    While the child prolongs a hum, encourage them to feel not only the vibration around the lips and face, but also to listen to the 'rounded' quality of the sound.

3   Vowel sounds can then be added to the hum, making sure that initially the focus remains on the hum rather than the vowel, to prevent any increase in glottal tension. The child may then be able to produce the hum with simultaneous onset of breath and voice. We feel that it is useful to allow the child to imitate a hum with a breathy onset, as well as a hum with a hard glottal onset and then hopefully they will be able to feel the difference when they try to produce a sound with simultaneous (gentle) onset.

    Try the following sounds:

    mmm ... ah   *mmm ... ay*
    mmm ... oo   *mmm ... oh*
    mmm ... ee   *mmm ... eye*

4   Once the child has mastered these, the clinician can move on to words and phrases, maintaining an intoned voice and initially prolonging the hum at the beginning of the words.

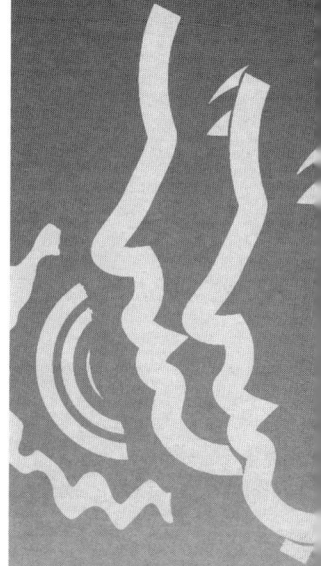

EXERCISES TO ESTABLISH THE HUMMING TECHNIQUE *(continued)*

Words

Main	Many
Mine	Money
Mean	Morning
Moan	Moaning
Moon	Mining
Mourn	Meaning

Short phrases

Many moons

Many more

Morn or noon

More money

My name

Many miles

Moaning Minnie

Manage money

Longer phrases

My name is Naomi More

My mum makes mince on Mondays

My money may go missing

Mad Max moans from morning till night

Noisy monkeys made away with it

Mean Mary mocks Mike

Many miles more to the mountain

Martin has marmalade in the morning

Mandy likes mince and minestrone soup

Easy Onset of Voice

The following exercises allow for easy coordination of airflow and voice, and are designed to counteract vocally abusive habits – for example, a hard glottal attack. By reducing the laryngeal and vocal tract tensions, it is possible to reduce the amount, and force of contact of the vocal folds.

When working with children using this technique, the clinician must ensure that the voice quality does not become too 'breathy', as this may lead to hypoadduction of the vocal folds at the posterior ends.

EXERCISES TO ESTABLISH EASY ONSET

1   Ask the child to breathe in gently, and then out on a *h*.

Repeat this several times, making sure that the child does not produce a
forced whisper, resulting in constriction of the vocal tract. If the child is unable
to produce a gentle sound without constriction, try using a rolled up piece of
paper, and when it is very tightly rolled up blow down the tube. Follow this
with blowing down a more loosely rolled piece of paper to demonstrate the
difference in the airflow.

2   Now ask the child to add some vowel sounds, listening carefully to the sound
to observe any tension:

h ... ah	*h ... ay*
h ... oo	*h ... oh*
h ... ee	*h ... eye*

3   Once this has been achieved, try the vowel sounds again, except with *s*, *f*
and *sh*.

4   Using the story of *Jack and the Beanstalk*, ask the child to say the part: 'Fe, fi,
fo, fum I smell an Englishman ...'.

5   Children also enjoy saying nonsense words, for example:

'shay, shoh, shee'
'sah, soh, sigh'
'foo, fay, fee'

6   The following word lists can be practised by the child. Remember to listen
carefully for any signs of tension creeping back in:

high	hoe	he	hay	who
hill	hail	hole	hell	heel
him	harm	home	whom	hum
horn	hen	hand	hound	hang

EXERCISES TO ESTABLISH EASY ONSET *(continued)*

say	sigh	see	sew	sue
sign	sin	seen	sane	sawn
soon	same	seam	sum	sing
sail	sell	sole	seal	sill
fail	file	fill	fell	foal
farm	fame	foam	phone	fine
fun	fan	fin	fawn	fang
shy	she	show	shoe	shear
shame	sheen	shine	shown	shone
share	shore	shell	shail	shoal

7   Have the child try the following contrasting words, making sure there is no
sign of a hard attack with those words that begin with a vowel sound:

hoe	oh	shame	aim
high	I	shy	eye
hill	ill	sheet	eat
hail	ale	shake	ache
his	is	share	air
hat	at	shout	out
hear	ear	sheer	ear
harm	arm	shark	ark
hold	old	shoulder	older
hand	and	show	oh
hedge	edge	shy	I

(Adapted from Martin & Darnley, 1992)

EXERCISES TO ESTABLISH EASY ONSET *(continued)*

8 When the child has mastered a gentle onset with vowel initial words, try some phrases such as:

All over again

Everyone over there

Are you angry?

I ate all the apples

I am an ostrich

I am an Eskimo

Uncle Arthur is amusing

I am all ears

Over and over and over again

For ever and ever and ever

Orange eggs at Easter

Ugly elephants are amusing

Playing 'Consequences' will help to reinforce these phrases. For example, each child could pick a word to make a sentence beginning with 'I am ...', an eagle, ostrich, egg, ambulance driver, ant, or early bird.

Chewing

This voice therapy technique can be rather fun to do with children, and can be extremely effective for releasing tension in the jaw and tongue. It is good for children with poor resonance and clarity. By releasing the tension in the tongue and jaw it allows the larynx to 'drop down' within the vocal tract, and the resulting phonation is similar to that produced in humming with strong oral/nasal resonance.

EXERCISES TO ESTABLISH THE TECHNIQUE OF CHEWING

1 Ideally, sit the child in front of a mirror to take advantage of visual feedback. Ask the child to pretend that they are chewing a large piece of toffee. With younger children, the clinician could use pictures of a cow 'chewing', or stories with which the child can join in.

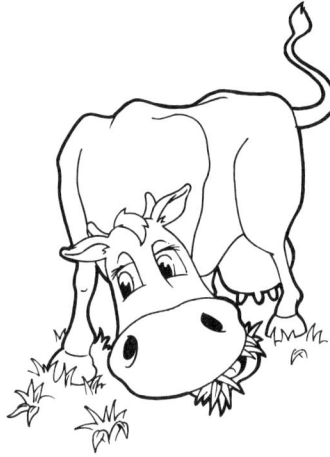

Encourage the child to chew in a relaxed, open-mouthed, exaggerated manner, making sure that they are incorporating large movements of their tongue as well as their jaw.

2 When they are chewing in a nice easy manner, ask them to try to produce the following vowel sounds:

ah ...oh ... ee ... oo   *ay ... eye ... oh ... ow*
oo ... ah ... ee ... ay   *ee ... ow ... oo ... oh*
oh ... ah ... eye ... ay   *eye ... oo ... ee ... ah*

If the child appears to be holding their tongue tightly in the back of their mouth, the sound 'yam' can be used (with a variety of vowel sounds in the middle). This encourages the tongue to continue to rise, fall and move forward during the exercise (Boone, 1980). Encourage the child to listen to the sound that is produced.

3 Once this has been achieved, try simultaneous chewing and voicing on the following phrases:

I am in   all alone
I am over   in awe
I am up   in or out
all over   under or over
all out   only an hour
over easy   arm in arm

Yawn-sigh

Yawning encourages opening and relaxing of the entire vocal tract, including lowering and relaxing the larynx. The yawn opens up the oral space; exercises the facial muscles; lifts the soft palate, and then releases the jaw. It is also one of the best ways in which to release tension in the pharynx. It is one of the most widely used techniques in adult voice therapy, in particular for patients with muscle tension dysphonia, as it results in minimal closure of the vocal folds, which become shorter and more lax. The sound produced is therefore usually slightly breathy.

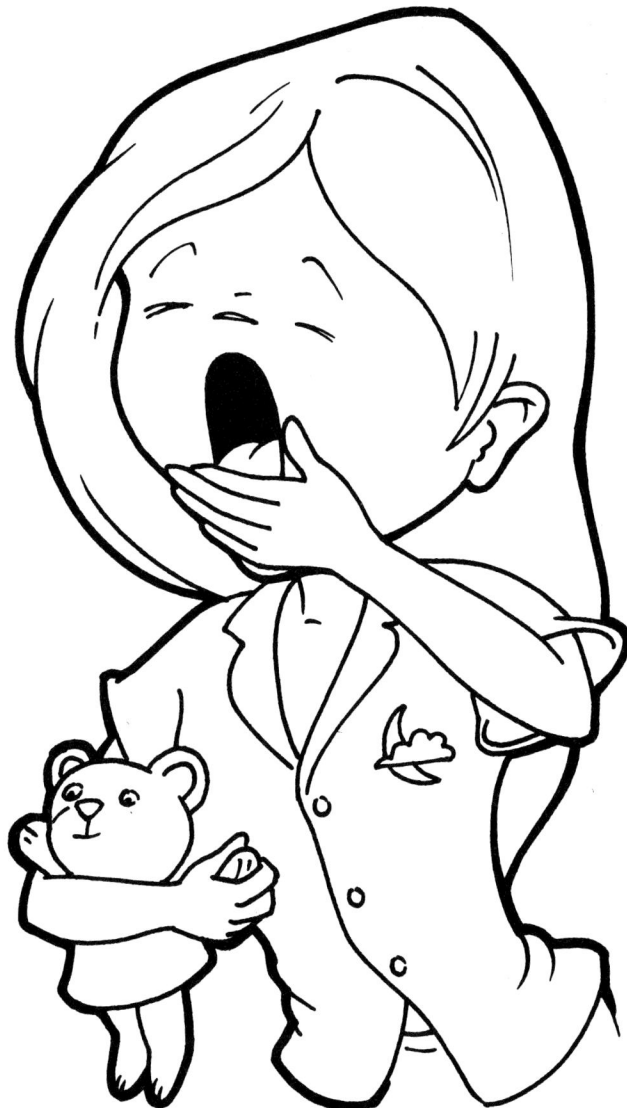

EXERCISES TO ESTABLISH YAWN-SIGH

1   Ask the child to open their mouth as wide as possible, and move into a yawn. If the child finds this difficult to do, then the clinician can demonstrate, and as yawns tend to be infectious, the child will usually follow suit! This can work very well in a group setting.

Encourage the child to practise some yawns on their own, being aware of the space created inside their mouth as the back of the tongue 'drops down'. Too much space between the upper and lower jaw will lead to excessive tension.

2   Now try some stifled yawns with the child, with the lips lightly closed. Ask the child whether they can feel their ears 'popping'.

3   From the yawn, ask the child to move into a sigh on expiration of the following vowels:

Yawn ... *oh*
Yawn ... *ay*
Yawn ... *ow*
Yawn ... *oo*
Yawn ... *eye*
Yawn ... *ah*
Yawn ... *ee*

Encourage the child to listen to the vocal tone of the open, relaxed pharynx, which contributes a mellow, full sound to the voice. As the child produces a pitch glide down, listen carefully to ensure that they do not produce any pitch breaks.

EXERCISES TO ESTABLISH YAWN-SIGH *(continued)*

4   Once the feeling of the yawn with the vowel sounds is established, try the following phrases using the same open, relaxed vocal tract:

oh no	half past	how now	name game
go home	Mark's car	loud howl	may rain
so slow	car park	bounce down	hay bale

do you	see me	my line
new moon	please eat	why wine
whose room	three bees	fly high

For younger children or non-readers, use pictures to reinforce some of the above phrases – for example, a snail for 'so slow', or some bumble bees for 'three bees'.

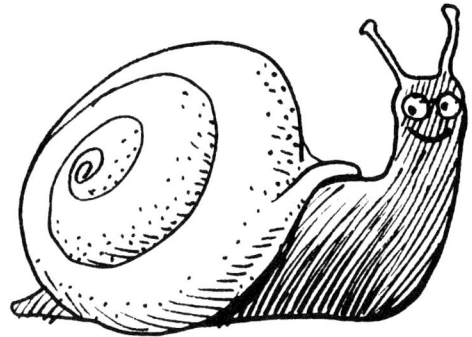

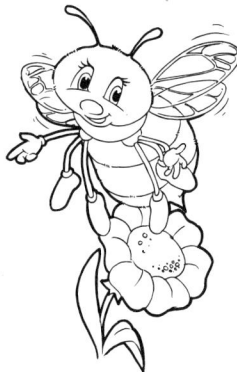

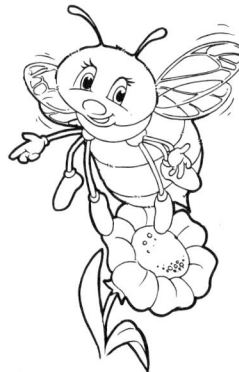

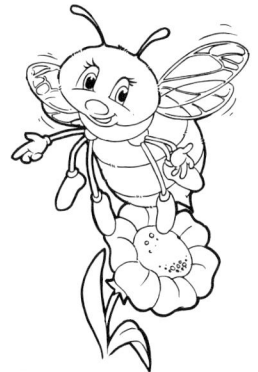

Ideas for Extending the Above Vocal Techniques

◆ 'Mr Men'-type stories: characters to include Mr Tired (always 'Yawning'), Mr Song (always 'Humming'), and Mr Hungry (always 'Chewing').

◆ Stories that include characters who evoke each voice therapy technique. For example, the Giant in *Jack and the Beanstalk* ('fee, fi, fo, fum ...'); the Wolf in the *Three Little Pigs* ('I'll huff and I'll puff ...').

Other Voice Therapy Techniques

In the authors' experience, all the above techniques can be used fairly successfully with children, although some modifications may need to be made in order to ensure that every child understands the exercises. There are other techniques, such as the Accent Method (Thyme-Frøkjær & Frøkjær-Jensen, 2001); Estill's Compulsory Figures; inhalation phonation, and glottal onset or forcing exercises (pushing/pulling), which could easily be adapted – particularly for older children. However, the authors have not had a great deal of experience in using these with dysphonic children. The *Voice Clinic Handbook* (Harris *et al*, 2000) contains excellent descriptions of these therapy techniques.

RESONANCE

The concept of resonance is one of the most difficult to communicate to dysphonic children. Therefore, prior to any work focused on this area of voice production, the clinician may need to spend a considerable amount of time ensuring the child has an understanding of what resonance is, and how it affects the quality of the voice.

Andrews (1986) uses storybook characters to personify the behavioural characteristics associated with the 'old' vocal pattern and the 'new', desirable, behaviour. For example, 'Wendy the Wicked Witch' contrasted with a beautiful princess.

Prior to starting any actual work on resonance, the child's posture and alignment must be correct, and there should be no obvious signs of tension in and around the vocal tract. Resonance is a feature of a number of languages, and may therefore be perceived differently by some cultural and ethnic groups (Martin & Lockhart, 2000), so consideration may need to be given to this when working with particular children.

ACTIVITIES TO ENCOURAGE AWARENESS OF RESONANCE

◆ Identifying the resonating cavities (mouth, nose, throat and chest). Use the pictures and diagrams from the anatomy exercises.

◆ Demonstrating how changes in the size and shape of these cavities may affect the sound of the voice (perhaps using characters such as the 'Wide Mouth Frog', or 'Karen with the chronic cold').

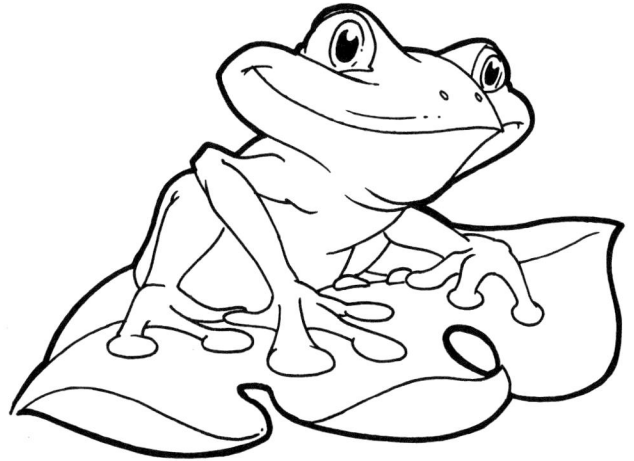

◆ Showing how tension in the vocal tract affects resonance. The clinician, for example speaking a sentence with a closed mouth or clenched jaw, can easily demonstrate this. Ask the children how the voice quality is affected, but perhaps give them some words to choose from – for example, rough, smooth, clear, quiet, tight.

◆ Explaining the difference between oral and nasal resonance, for example /m/ and /a/.

The aim of therapy is to achieve appropriate, or balanced, resonance in the child's spoken voice – often referred to as the 'tone focus'.

Encouraging Oral Resonance

Start by encouraging an open mouth posture for connected speech, in order to enhance oral resonance, which will also result in opening the pharynx, lifting the soft palate, and lowering the larynx. Sentences such as the ones below, with non-oral pressure consonants, require increased air pressure in the mouth. It can sometimes be helpful for the child to start by saying each phrase with very little, or minimal, oral movement in order to feel and hear the difference.

Sentences to encourage oral resonance:

> Kick the ball over the wall.
> Pick the apple, pick the pear.
> The ditch is wide, adjust your stride.
> Twitch, hop, plop, the rabbit has stopped.
> Pit-a-pat, what is that?
> Eight fat cats sat by the rat.
> Theresa baked pies with peas.
> > (Andrews, 1986)

Rhymes such as 'Pat-a-cake, pat-a-cake baker's man…' can be used to reinforce the above with younger children.

Phrases beginning with open vowels will encourage mouth opening, and may help to reduce nasality if needed.

Phrases with open vowels:

> Apple pie is good
> Often enough
> All right with me
> Odd couple
> End of the line
> Eggs and toast

Ever see one?

Only a little late

Up and down

After you

Encouraging Nasal Resonance

Humming is an excellent way to encourage nasal resonance, and is often quite easy for children, as they can feel the vibration around the top of the lips and down the nose. As before, start with a gentle but resonant hum on its own, followed by a smooth transition into vowel sounds, and then into words and phrases (see above).

Children with dysphonia often present with weak or thin resonance, which means that the voice lacks richness and carrying power. Chanting is frequently effective in creating kinaesthetic and auditory awareness of increased resonance in the oral and nasal cavities. The following phrases should be practised with prolonged vowels, and where possible the child's attention should be drawn to the 'sound carrying' consonants (voiced continuants), as well as encouraging them to use an open mouth posture and to exaggerate lip movement.

Sentences to encourage nasal resonance:

Rosie revs the engine.

Beams zoom towards the moon.

Hey ho, Hey ho, they are all dwarfs you know.

The treasure is golden coins, rubies, emeralds.

(Andrews 1986)

Once the child can produce the above sentences with appropriate resonance, it is worth trying a few more sentences with balanced phonemes, incorporating both oral and nasal resonance.

Sentences to encourage oral and nasal resonance:

I don't feel well.

Is it lunchtime?

Do you know her?

Can you reach that?

Don't open the window.

Please turn on the TV.

The cat climbed the tree.

He ran around the lake.

Give the book to him.

The children made lots of noise.

PITCH AND VOCAL FLEXIBILITY

In Chapter 2, it was mentioned that children have a limited range of options to use in order to vary their voice, and they often become habituated to only one strategy, such as increasing volume in order to either gain or hold someone's attention. Therefore, an essential part of voice therapy with children is to enable them to use other vocal options, such as pitch and vocal flexibility.

Pitch work can be great fun with children, and working to improve pitch flexibility often lessens the strain on the larynx.

ACTIVITIES TO EXPLORE PITCH AND FLEXIBILITY

1   Use musical instruments to demonstrate changes in pitch.

2   Improve awareness of pitch changes by telling stories such as 'Little Red Riding Hood', with one character (Grandma) who has a deep voice, and one (Little Red Riding Hood) who has a quiet, gentle and high-pitched voice.

3   Sing up and down a scale with the child, either with a hum or sung with a *lah*. Use spatial cues, such as going up and down a ladder, or use a hand to manipulate an imaginary yo-yo.

4   In a group setting, make up a story with different noises with which the children can join in. The story could contain wolves, or the wind going *woo*, or an ambulance going *ng-ah*.

5   Use contrastive pairs of words to encourage movement between high and low pitch. It is often easier for the child to do these in a 'sing-song' voice:

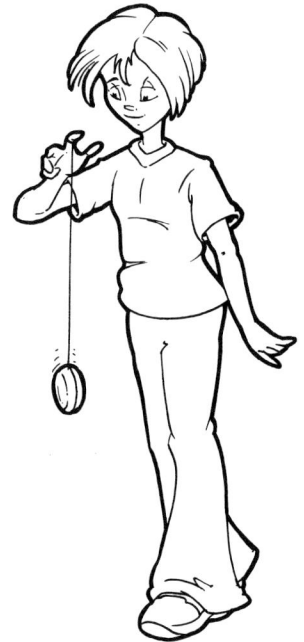

HIGH	LOW
ping	pong
ding	dong
high	low
hill	valley
sky	sea
jump	dive
up	down
soft	hard
top	bottom
fun	work

(Martin & Darnley, 1992)

ACTIVITIES TO EXPLORE PITCH AND FLEXIBILITY *(continued)*

This can work well within a group setting, where children can bob up and down along with the changes in pitch – perhaps stretching high or crouching down low – so long as they are able to retain reasonable posture and breath support.

6   Using words that encourage either high or low pitch to be associated with their meaning can also help vocal flexibility. Say the words first, then ask the child to say whether they think it should be a high or a low sound, again using the bobbing up and down game along with the words:

HIGH	LOW
squeal	dungeon
creak	dark
cheep	gloomy
fly	sink
shrill	deep
tingle	grumble
yelp	grunt
sing	thump
flitter	groan
hiss	boo

(Martin & Darnley, 1992)

7   Move on to sentences to show pitch variety:

I zipped my jacket up and down.

The submarine sank to the bottom of the sea.

The roller coaster goes up and down.

I'll climb up and then look down at you.

Surprise, surprise! Happy Birthday.

The drum went 'boom, boom, boom'.

The cat gave a squeak and slid under my bed.

The tiny kitten climbed to the very top of the tree.

Deep in the forest, the girl was lost.

The ball bounced up and up into the net.

The man had a gruff and angry voice.

She laughed and laughed with happiness.

(Andrews, 1986)

8   Give older children sentences to read aloud in several different emotions, for example in happy, sad, bored, or excited voices:

My mum has won the lottery!

I shall be leaving soon.

Please can we go to the party?

I will have to do it all over again.

Vocal Flexibility

A greater range and flexibility of individual muscle groups within the vocal apparatus helps to prevent strain or damage to the larynx. This area must be handled sensitively by the clinician, as cultural considerations should be recognised, and it is the norm for older children to have very limited muscularity. The clinician must emphasise that over-exaggerated movements are essential for practising the exercises, and that it is hoped that these will carry over into connected speech with minimal effort.

The authors feel that it is useful to begin with some of the following exercises to 'free up' the muscles.

ACTIVITIES TO ENCOURAGE MUSCULAR FLEXIBILITY

1 Jaw

◆ Have the child clench the jaw, with teeth pressed together. Now they should relax, and feel the difference between the tension and release.

◆ Have the child open the mouth wide and feel the space created between the back teeth. Ask the child to put their fingers flat over the temperomandibular joint. Make sure that there is no 'bunching' of the muscle.

◆ Have the child move their jaw from side to side.

◆ Have the child rotate their jaw in a figure of eight. Then move it in the other direction.

◆ A relaxed open yawn is a good way of increasing jaw muscularity, and is a very effective way of releasing tension.

◆ Massage the jaw muscles from the 'hinge' down.

2 Lips

◆ Have the child keep their lips lightly together, and chew an imaginary piece of toffee. Monitor tension levels, as initially there can be a feeling of discomfort at the temporomandibular joint.

◆ Ask the child to purse their lips and rotate them in a clockwise direction. This should be repeated several times, and then the lip contact released, before doing it again in the opposite direction.

◆ With their lips closed, the child should blow air into the cheeks, and hold it for about five seconds. Press their fingers against the cheeks, in order to 'pop' them, allowing the air to escape.

◆ Tell the child to maintain light contact between the lips, purse and then spread them into a smile, feeling the contrasting muscle activity in the lips and cheeks.

◆ The child should blow out through the lips, rather as a horse does, so that the lips vibrate very rapidly. Encourage them to feel the movement in their lips, and the residual tingling.

ACTIVITIES TO ENCOURAGE MUSCULAR FLEXIBILITY *(continued)*

3 Tongue

◆ Practising chewing again. This time the child should move their tongue around inside the mouth, as if trying to move the toffee from one side to the other, and then from front to back.

◆ With the tip of their tongue, they should gently 'massage' the back molar on the top left-hand side for about 20 seconds. This should be repeated on all of the other back molars.

◆ Tell the child to imagine that there is food stuck between the teeth and the upper and lower lips, and to lick around and over the surfaces of the teeth for about 20 seconds.

◆ Ask the child to extend the tip of their tongue outside the mouth as far as possible (this will stretch the tongue base). Then they move it from side to side and up and down.

4 Pharynx

◆ Keeping the lips lightly together, the child should try to produce a full or stifled yawn, feeling the space that is created at the back of the mouth.

◆ Ask the child to try to deliberately create tension in the jaw, tongue and pharynx while counting or saying the days of the week. Then try practising without the tension, and notice the difference in the voice quality.

Increasing Muscular Flexibility within Speech

Once awareness, control and flexibility of the articulators have been achieved, it is important to encourage the child to carry this over into connected speech. It is essential that the child understands that by allowing greater flexibility of their articulation, their voice will also improve, because they will be able to achieve emphasis, clarity and carrying power without straining the vocal apparatus.

Using tongue twisters, which most children love, is an excellent way to encourage greater articulatory flexibility. As the child says the following tongue twisters, try to make them more meaningful by acting them out, or clapping or stamping out the rhythm:

A big beetle bit a body in a big black bag.

The monkey munched melon and macaroni.

A sick sparrow sang six sad songs.

A crow flew over the river with a lump of raw liver.

Five French friars fanning a fainted flee.

Cheerful children chant charming tunes.

A thin little boy picked six thick thistle sticks.

A king carried crates of cabbages across a crooked court.

(Andrews, 1986)

Chapter 9: The Group Approach to Therapy and Therapy Evaluation

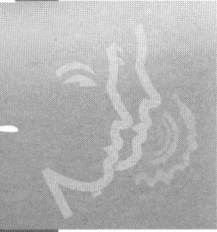

INTRODUCTION

The establishment of the authors' children's voice group as an effective way of working with childhood dysphonia came from two clinicians combining their expertise. One of the authors was a senior community clinician, struggling to provide effective therapy to children with voice problems. The other was a senior clinician in an acute hospital with a developing specialism in voice disorders. One colleague contacted the other for specialist advice, which, although it was sound advice, needed 'translation' for the paediatric case-load. Group therapy was already an established and proven method of working with a variety of children's communication problems, and with dysphonic adults, and by combining the professional skills of the authors, the children's voice group was established. At the same time, the awareness of voice disorders for all clinicians in the service was raised as a result of the setting up of a combined voice clinic at the hospital with the otolaryngologist, and an increase in identified voice problems ensued.

MODEL OF CARE

When developing any model or programme of care, clinicians need to ensure that the system is flexible enough for it to be accessed at any point. Children's voice problems may develop gradually over a number of years, and parents often report that a voice has 'always sounded like that'. This makes it very difficult for anyone other than a trained listener to detect a voice problem, unless the child becomes aphonic. As a result, the child's voice problem is usually detected by a clinician when the child attends an appointment for an unrelated problem, such as dysfluency or immature phonology. This is the most usual route to voice therapy. Very occasionally, if, for example, the problem occurs suddenly following an attack of laryngitis, parents or guardians may take their child to the GP. Ideally, the next step, whatever the first contact, is a referral to a combined voice clinic (Figure 6). An accurate diagnosis is essential if later therapy is to be effective.

The initial assessment, outlined in Chapter 3, may be carried out by the community clinician prior to the voice clinic appointment, or afterwards by the clinicians who run the treatment groups. If possible, all community clinicians should be skilled in

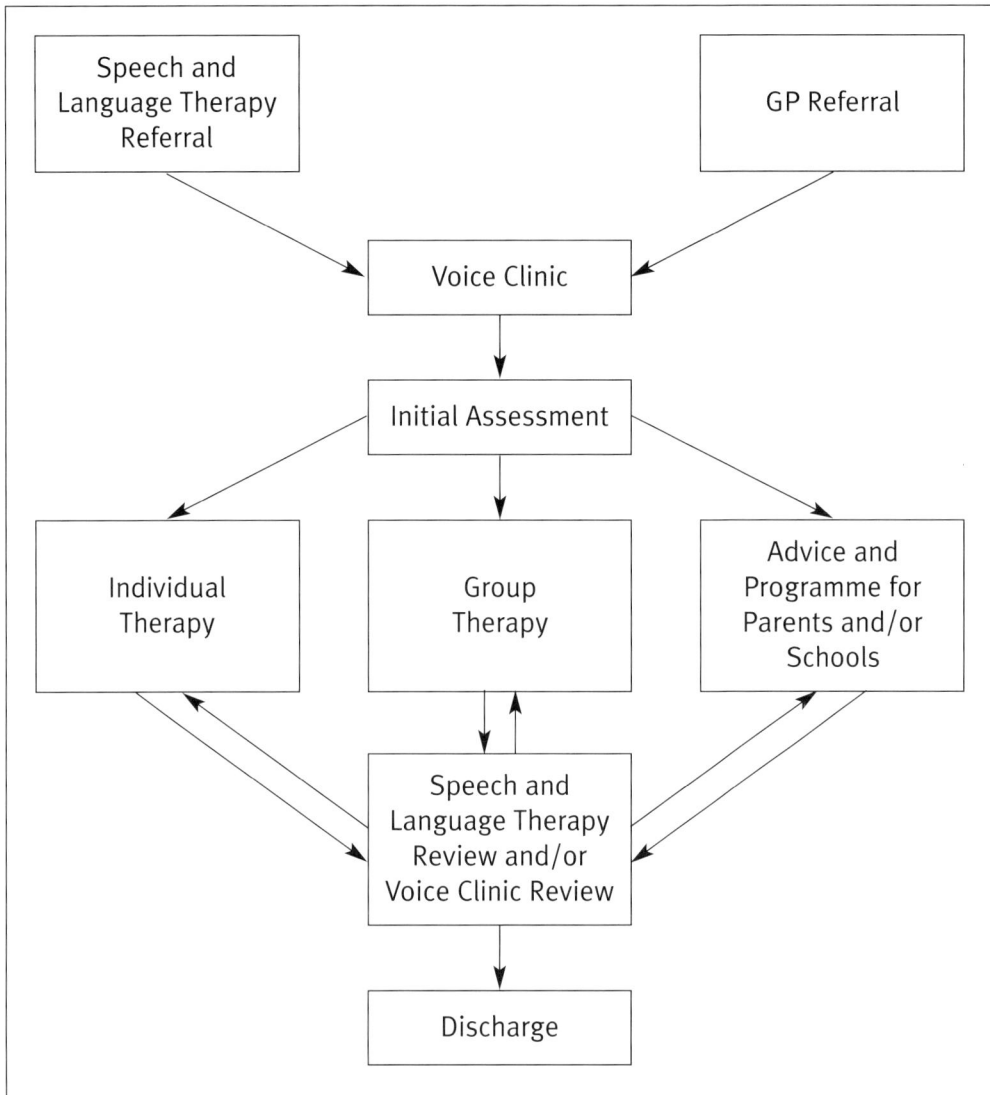

Figure 6 Model of Care: Dysphonic Children

carrying out the assessment, so that the number of assessment appointments for the child and their family are kept to a minimum.

When both these assessments have been completed, the clinician must then make a decision as to the type of appropriate intervention. Some of the factors to be taken into account at this point are discussed in Chapter 4. Although the authors' experience indicates that group therapy is the most effective intervention option, it should not be viewed as the only option, as using programmes at home or attending for individual therapy can also achieve results.

Working with dysphonic children is not usually a 'quick fix' option, and it is essential that the child and family are aware that therapy may take months and, on occasion, years. This is due to the multiplicity of contributing factors (Chapter 2), and the inherent difficulties of altering and adapting vocal behaviour in a potentially unmotivated child.

As a result, the child can be in the cycle of therapy, voice clinic reviews and speech and language therapy reviews for some time. Families will need to be supported throughout this process in order to maintain motivation, and one of the clinician's primary roles is to highlight any vocal improvements. These advances are likely to be gradual, and therefore the child and parents are often unable to detect that the voice has improved at all.

GROUP ADMINISTRATION

Appendix 9 is included for use by clinicians in community clinics wanting to set up and run a children's voice group. The voice modification programme (Appendix 5) and supporting star chart (Appendix 6) are used with all children who have a voice problem.

In order to maintain good communication with the combined voice clinic at the hospital, brief status reports are sent following each run of groups, and after every speech and language therapy review. This ensures that, no matter when the Consultant Otolaryngologist reviews the child, they are always aware of the current situation and the child's progress to date.

MEASURING OUTCOMES

Ramig and Verdolini (1998) stress the importance of measuring an individual's social function, because voice disorders affect self-image and can impact on individuals both socially and economically – for example, a school teacher. They refer to the use of World Health Organisation classifications of disease (WHO, 1980) in this context. These call for measurement of impact on the individual and on the individual's social function, alongside measurement of the severity of the actual disease.

Pannbacker (1998) is one of many authors highlighting the need for more research on the efficacy of voice treatments, but she lists several problems with the establishment of such research:

Problems with establishing data on efficacy of treatment
◆ Differences in aetiology of voice problems
◆ Small numbers of subjects
◆ Inadequate information about nature and severity of the voice problems
◆ Lack of appropriate control groups
◆ Failure to report frequency, extent and/or duration of treatment
◆ Absence of long-term follow-up evaluations
◆ Lack of information about subjects such as gender.

In 1997, Verdolini, *et al* reviewed all the efficacy studies on voice therapy, decade by decade, beginning in the 1940s. In that decade the only studies were on the following:

1 Expression of expert opinion
2 The claim that therapy works at all
3 One retrospective study with a control group.

Between 1990 and 1996, the depth and range of studies were considerably increased as shown below:

Range of efficacy studies
1 True experimental studies predominate.
2 Double-blind placebo-controlled studies appear.
3 Functional, 'quality of life' issues surface more strongly.
4 Client/clinician interface addressed.
5 Instrumental variables studied in relation to final variables.
6 Learning and compliance become formal topics.
7 Cross-study investigations are conducted.
8 Theory-based models of voice therapy are developed.
9 Database study reported.

Although many of the findings from this review of over five decades of research apply solely to the adult case-load – for example those relating to Parkinson's Disease – other conclusions are relevant to all voice problems:

Research findings on the impact of voice therapy

1 Functional aphonias can sometimes be successfully treated with the use of facilitatory, vegetative voicing manouevres.

2 Conventional voice therapy and resonant voice therapy may produce benefits in the treatment of nodules, beyond benefits seen for hygiene intervention alone.

3 Voice efficiency may improve with a vocal function exercise programme.

4 Loudness reduction may be facilitated by the use of a behavioural programme including positive reinforcement and aversive stimulation, at least in a cognitively impaired individual.

5 Voice therapy is a useful and important topic of investigation, given reports of functional impairments and disruptions to quality of life subsequent to voice problems.

Since the focus of this review is weighted towards adult clients, it may be appropriate to substitute 'cognitively impaired individual' (number four) with an individual not yet having fully developed cognition.

MEASURING OUTCOMES IN CLINICS

As mentioned in Chapter 4 above, it is essential to set appropriate therapy aims, some of which may not include any notion of a 'cure'. An appropriate aim, agreed with the child and their parents or guardians, can aid motivation as they witness the aim becoming a reality. The achievement of an aim, however small, can provide the necessary motivation for tackling the next step.

Measuring step-by-step goals not only facilitates monitoring of the progress of therapy, but also enables both the goals and the therapy to be adapted as circumstances change. Measuring overall outcomes validates the therapy process, and in so doing can add to the existing body of clinical evidence that is vital in informing clinical practice. The use of simple but effective outcome measurements can, in this way, support the clinical governance structure of a service where there is limited time or resources to implement research projects.

The authors have used an adapted version (Hunt & Slater, 1999) of WHO-Enderby *Therapy Outcome Measures* (Enderby, 1997) in their clinical work, and have found these are also suited to the paediatric dysphonic case-load. Clinicians may wish to use other models for measuring outcomes, the discussion of which is not within the remit of this book. Clinicians wishing to explore other options may find Carding (2000), and Martin and Lockhart (2000) useful sources for reference.

For clinicians familiar with WHO-Enderby *Therapy Outcome Measures*, the record sheet (Appendix 4) enables a comparison of duration, frequency and method of therapy, for children having the same diagnosis and the same initial impairment score. The information is collated once the child has been discharged on successful completion of therapy. Figure 7 gives examples of the kind of information available to the clinician using these record sheets. The charts show that group therapy is more effective than individual therapy, particularly when there is a more severe impairment rating (2).

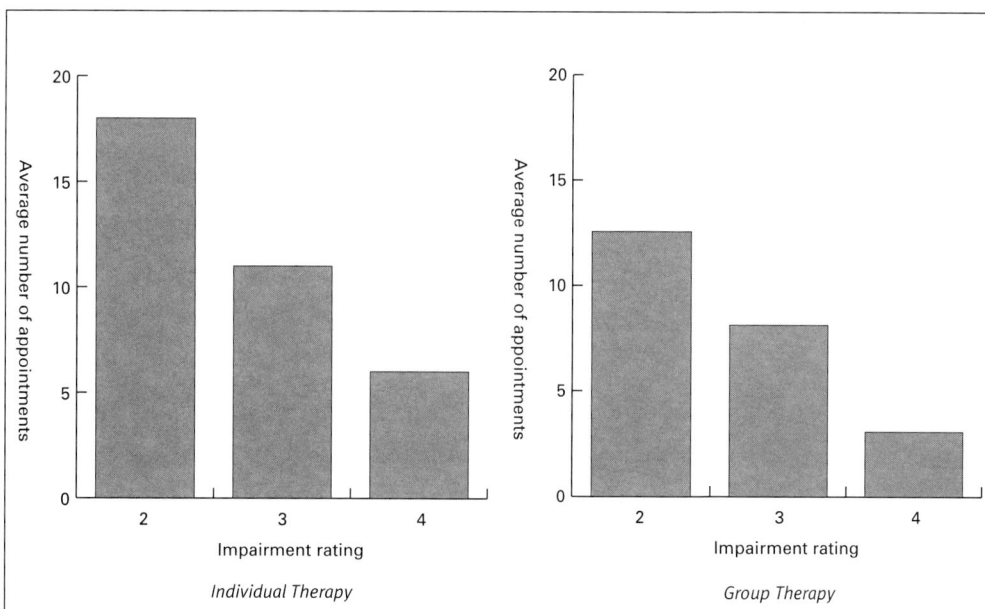

Figure 7
Examples of Information Collated from Therapy Outcome Measures (sample = 147)

CHILDREN WHO MAY NOT RESPOND

It is essential that a clinician is honest both with the parents or guardians, and the child when therapy is not being successful, rather than trying until all motivation is lost. If the timing of the original intervention, for whatever reason, is inappropriate, it may be that, following a complete break from therapy lasting several months, results can be achieved at a later date. The following list outlines some of the reasons for unsuccessful interventions that have occurred in the authors' experience:

◆ Poor motivation to change vocal habits (Case Summary 5, pp31–32)
◆ Learning difficulties
◆ Other structural defects – for example, a cleft palate
◆ Children with English as a second language
◆ Additional medical problems, such as asthma or a hearing impairment
◆ General immaturity
◆ Misdiagnosis, such as a missed micro-web, resulting in inappropriate therapy.

In these cases, the professional credibility of the clinician is enhanced by an honest acknowledgement that no improvement can be made, whereas continuous and ineffective therapy devalues the profession for clients and fellow professionals alike.

SUMMARY

The authors firmly believe that the group approach to therapy is the most effective way of resolving childhood dysphonia (Hunt & Slater, 1995). Nevertheless, the decision to treat in a group or individually is not a question of a 'right' or 'wrong' choice, as both are valid options. Whichever route the clinician chooses to take, the success of any intervention remains the prime objective. However, unless these successes are recorded, with the use of robust outcome measures that allow for the evaluation of therapy, evidence-based practice will not develop. Professionally, it is necessary for clinicians to build up a body of evidence to support clinical practice and inform future therapy.

Appendixes

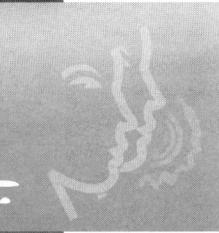

APPENDIX 1 – PAEDIATRIC VOICE CASE HISTORY

BIOGRAPHICAL INFORMATION

Name _____

Address _____

Tel no _____ Date of birth _____

Age _____ Age on assessment _____

Consultant Otolaryngologist _____

GP _____

Hospital no _____

Speech & Language Therapist _____

School/Nursery _____

Referral date _____ Date seen _____

ONSET AND HISTORY OF VOICE PROBLEM

Onset – gradual/sudden/present since child began speaking

Variation – home/school, intermittent/consistent, periods of complete loss

Sensory symptoms – coughing/throat-clearing, dry throat, pain, soreness, discomfort, ache

Parent's evaluation – thoughts on possible causal/contributory factors, effects of voice problem on child and family

APPENDIX 1 – PAEDIATRIC VOICE CASE HISTORY *(continued)*

VOICE USE/MISUSE

Home

Siblings

School

Other – singing, choir, drama, sports/strenuous exercise

Noise/surroundings

Personality type/how the voice is used – gaining and holding attention

FAMILY

History of voice problems in family

Awareness of stress/worries of child at home or school

APPENDIX 1 – PAEDIATRIC VOICE CASE HISTORY *(continued)*

SIGNIFICANT MEDICAL HISTORY

Developmental milestones

General health/appetite/size/weight

Sleeping patterns

Frequent coughs/colds/blocked nose

Hospitalisations – neonatal treatment, respiratory problems at birth, intubation, feeding problems.

Hearing loss

Irritants/environmental factors

smoke	YES / NO
hay fever	YES / NO
allergies	YES / NO
dry/dusty atmospheres	YES / NO
central heating	YES / NO
spicy foods	YES / NO
Mouth-breather?	YES / NO
Hydration/drinks	YES / NO

APPENDIX 2 – PERCEPTUAL VOICE EVALUATION

Posture (including head position):

Tension (General body/shoulder/neck):

Articulation:

VOICE EVALUATION

Pitch　　　　　　　　Appropriate ☐　High ☐　Low ☐　Unstable ☐

Pitch range　　　　　Appropriate ☐　Wide range ☐　Narrow range ☐

Intensity　　　　　　Appropriate ☐　Loud ☐　Quiet ☐　Unstable ☐

Breath support　　　Diaphragmatic ☐　Clavicular ☐　Abdominal ☐

Rate　　　　　　　　Appropriate ☐　Fast ☐　Slow ☐

Resonance　　　　　Appropriate ☐　Hyponasal ☐　Hypernasal ☐
　　　　　　　　　　　Audible nasal escape ☐　Cul-de-sac ☐　Thin ☐

Supralaryngeal tension　Absent/lax ☐　Moderate ☐　Severe ☐

Laryngeal tension　　Absent/lax ☐　Moderate ☐　Severe ☐

Phonation　　　　　Modal ☐　Harsh ☐　Breathy ☐　Creaky (fry) ☐
　　　　　　　　　　　Falsetto ☐

Severity of dysphonia　Mild ☐　Moderate ☐　Severe ☐

Other features　　　Pitch breaks ☐　Phonation breaks ☐
　　　　　　　　　　　Glottal attack ☐

Sensory symptoms　Pain ☐　Ache ☐　Soreness ☐　Dryness ☐
　　　　　　　　　　　Burning ☐

APPENDIX 2 – PERCEPTUAL VOICE EVALUATION *(continued)*

COMMENTS

LARYNGEAL FINDINGS

Indirect laryngoscopy

Stroboscopy

Direct larngoscopy

Review period

MANAGEMENT/RECOMMENDATIONS

Advice leaflet   YES / NO

Star chart initiated   YES / NO

Review period:

Name of therapist _____

Signature _____

APPENDIX 3 – VOICE CLINIC INFORMATION LEAFLET

This leaflet has been devised to help you understand why your child has been referred to the Voice Clinic and what to expect.

Why has your child been referred?

Your child's Speech & Language Therapist or Doctor has requested an appointment for you to be seen in our Voice Clinic.

The reason for the referral is usually to gain more information on the nature of your child's voice problem, and to plan an appropriate management programme.

What is a Voice Clinic?

A Voice Clinic is a combined clinic run jointly by a Consultant Otolaryngologist and a Speech & Language Therapist with specialist skills in voice disorders.

The aims of our clinic are as follows:

◆ To ensure an accurate diagnosis.

◆ To devise an appropriate management plan.

◆ To monitor your child's progress with their voice.

What to expect

1   Initially, the Consultant and the Speech & Language Therapist will question you in depth about your child's voice problem, and discuss any intervention or treatment that they may already have had.

2   Following this, the Consultant will examine your child, starting with the nose, moving on to the mouth, and then using an angled mirror to attempt to examine your child's voice box, including their vocal folds.

Some children find it difficult to tolerate the mirror at the back of the mouth. If this is the case, the Consultant will spray the child's throat with a small amount of anaesthetic to make it easier and more comfortable.

If you can, try to reassure your child that this will not hurt, but that it may feel a little uncomfortable.

3   Your child may then undergo further investigations, all of which are painless. These include another kind of examination called rigid laryngoscopy with stroboscopy or a fibre-optic nasendoscopy. Both of these instruments may be attached to a camera, so that the movement of your child's vocal folds can be captured on video.

4   The Consultant and the Speech & Language Therapist will then discuss their findings with you, and you will have time to ask further questions.

5   Your child may then be referred to the Speech and Language Therapy department (if they are not already under their care). You will usually be asked to bring your child back to the Voice Clinic for monitoring of their voice. It is quite rare for children to need any surgical intervention, but should this be necessary the Otolaryngologist will discuss this with you.

6   You will be given an advice sheet (if you have not already had one) to enable you to understand the nature of your child's voice problem, and what you can do in order to help.

If you are at all concerned about this appointment, or have any further questions, please do not hesitate to contact us.

We look forward to meeting you and your child in the Voice Clinic.

_____   _____

Consultant Otolaryngologist   Speech & Language Therapist

APPENDIX 4 – FORM FOR WHO-ENDERBY THERAPY OUTCOME MEASURES

SPEECH AND LANGUAGE THERAPY SERVICE

Clinic _____

CLINICAL EVALUATION USING WHO-ENDERBY

Name _____ Patient number _____

Diagnosis _____ Date of birth _____

LONG-TERM AIM(S)

Age _____

Start date _____ Discharge date _____

Number of sessions offered _____ Number attended _____

Aim(s) achieved   YES/NO   Variance factor _____

	Start	Predicted	Outcome
Impairment			
Disability			
Handicap			
Distress			
Agreement			

Variance factors

A   Environmental, emotional, social

B   Medical

C   Attendance

Di Carer compliance

Dii Client compliance

E   Service availability

F   Additional impairments (cognition/memory)

G   Inappropriate aim

APPENDIX 4 – FORM FOR WHO-ENDERBY THERAPY OUTCOME MEASURES *(continued)*

SHORT-TERM AIM 1

Start date _____ Target date _____ Achieved Y / N

Variance factor(s) _____

Number of sessions offered _____ Number attended _____

Advice/Training ☐   Individual ☐   Group ☐

SHORT-TERM AIM 2

Start date _____ Target date _____ Achieved Y / N

Variance factor(s) _____

Number of sessions offered _____ Number attended _____

Advice/Training ☐   Individual ☐   Group ☐

SHORT-TERM AIM 3

Start date _____ Target date _____ Achieved Y / N

Variance factor(s) _____

Number of sessions offered _____ Number attended _____

Advice/Training ☐   Individual ☐   Group ☐

APPENDIX 4 – FORM FOR WHO-ENDERBY THERAPY OUTCOME MEASURES *(continued)*

CONTINUATION SHEET   **Patient number** _____

SHORT-TERM AIM

Start date _____ Target date _____ Achieved Y / N

Variance factor(s) _____

Number of sessions offered _____ Number attended _____

Advice/Training ☐   Individual ☐   Group ☐

SHORT-TERM AIM

Start date _____ Target date _____ Achieved Y / N

Variance factor(s) _____

Number of sessions offered _____ Number attended _____

Advice/Training ☐   Individual ☐   Group ☐

SHORT-TERM AIM

Start date _____ Target date _____ Achieved Y / N

Variance factor(s) _____

Number of sessions offered _____ Number attended _____

Advice/Training ☐   Individual ☐   Group ☐

APPENDIX 5 – VOICE MODIFICATION PROGRAMME

ENCOURAGING BETTER USE OF VOICE IN CHILDREN

This programme will be accompanied by a star chart, which should be filled in regularly to give the child visual feedback on progress. All of these activities will be explained by, and practised with, the clinician.

1   VOICE REST

a   This should be a set period of time, once or twice a day (depending on circumstances). The length of voice rest will be agreed with the clinician.

b   An ideal time for voice rest is during a quiet activity – for example, watching television or reading.

2   THINGS TO AVOID

a   Shouting, screaming or loud laughing – for example, in the playground, during PE or playing with friends.

b   Singing or humming – for example, with music or in school concerts.

c   Raising voice over background noise – such as in the car, over other speakers, or against television.

d   Whispering.

e   Habitual coughing or throat-clearing (unless, of course, the child has a cold).

f   Hard attack.

3   THINGS TO ENCOURAGE

a   Use of gesture or mime during voice rest.

b   Putting hand up in class without a noisy intake of breath.

c   Gaining attention – for example, in PE or the playground, by clapping or tapping someone on the shoulder.

APPENDIX 5 – VOICE MODIFICATION PROGRAMME *(continued)*

    d   Walking over to a person, rather than shouting across a room, or playground, or upstairs.

    e   Good posture (standing or sitting) when talking.

4   SELF-MONITORING

Attendance at the group will reinforce the child's understanding and awareness of the difference between loud voice, whisper, and gentle voice. Use of a gentle voice should be encouraged in:

    a   Talking one-to-one

    b   Talking in a small group

    c   Reading aloud

    d   Talking at meal times

Having good models at home and school will also help the child. This might mean no raised voices and taking turns in conversations, thus preventing verbal competition and a battleground situation arising.

If there are any queries, please contact:

Speech & Language Therapist

APPENDIX 6 – VOICE STAR CHART

REWARD!

Have you tried to ...		Week 1	Week 2	Week 3	Week 4
Rest your voice					
Use good posture and breathing					
Avoid shouting					
Avoid coughing and throat-clearing					
Avoid hard attacks					
Avoid whispering					

APPENDIX 7 – LARGE STAR CHART PICTURES

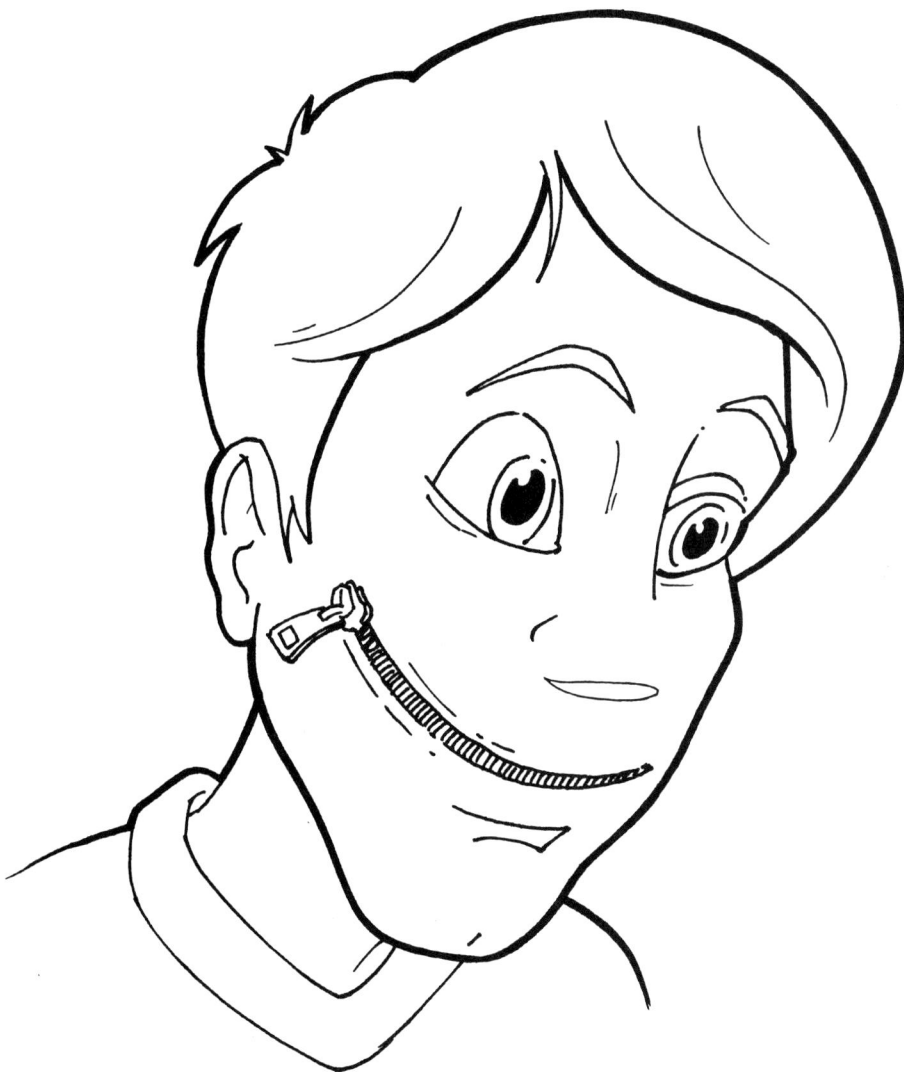

REST YOUR VOICE

APPENDIX 7 – LARGE STAR CHART PICTURES (continued)

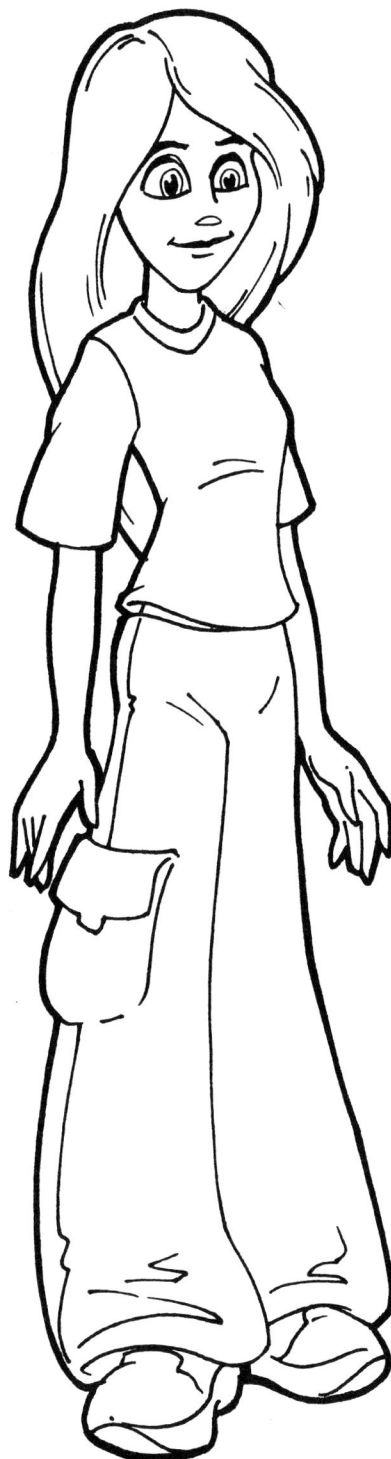

USE GOOD POSTURE AND BREATHING

132

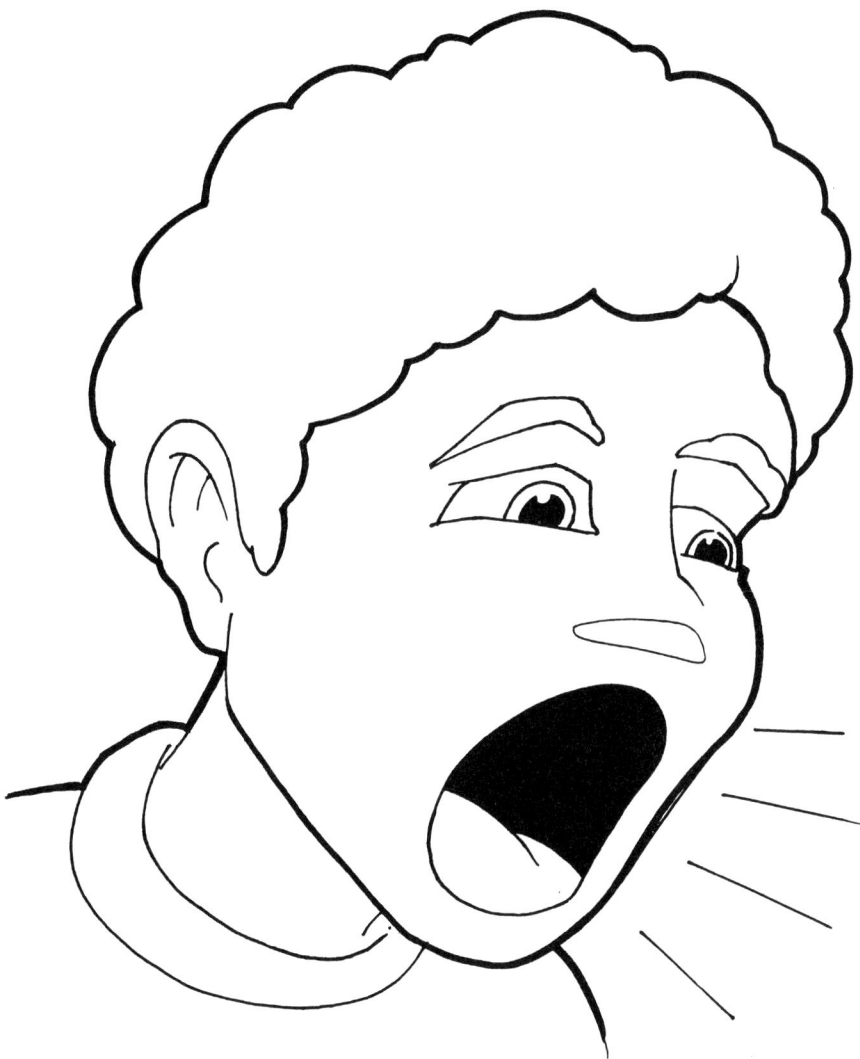

AVOID SHOUTING

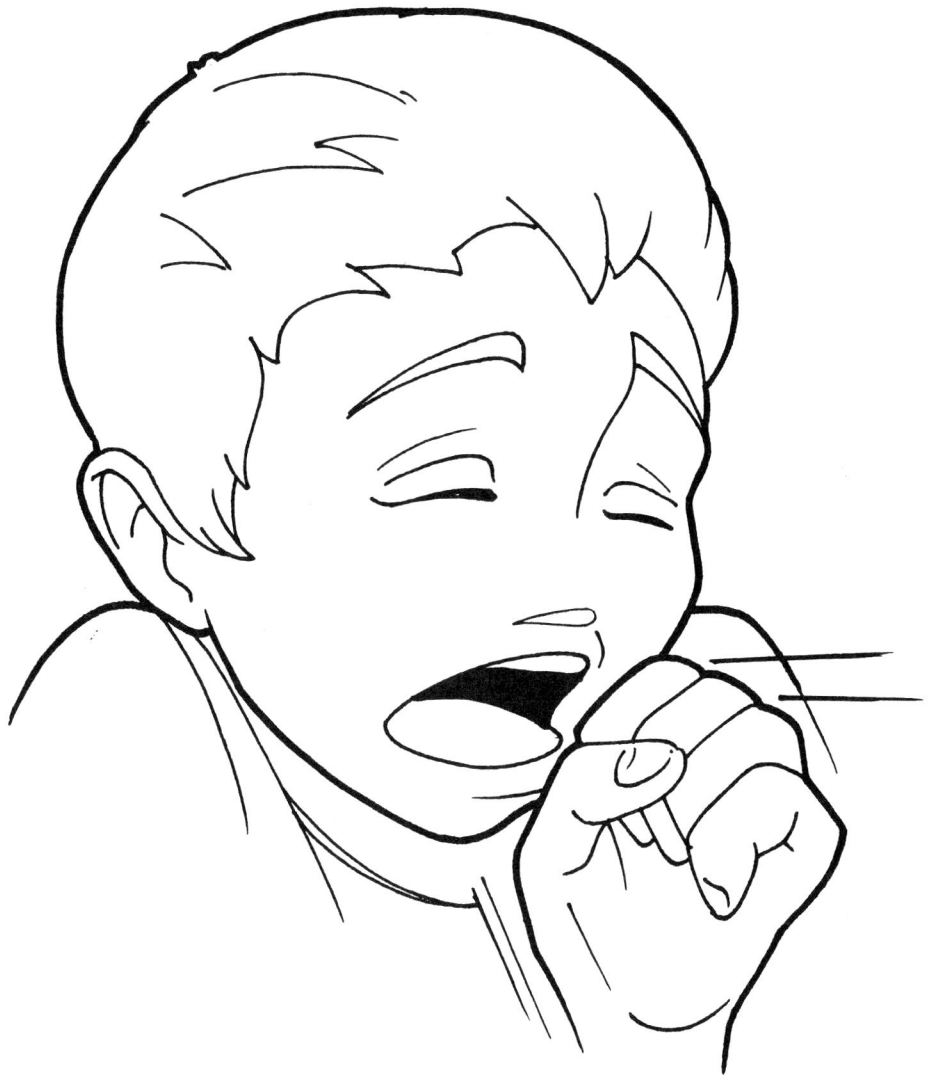

AVOID COUGHING AND THROAT-CLEARING

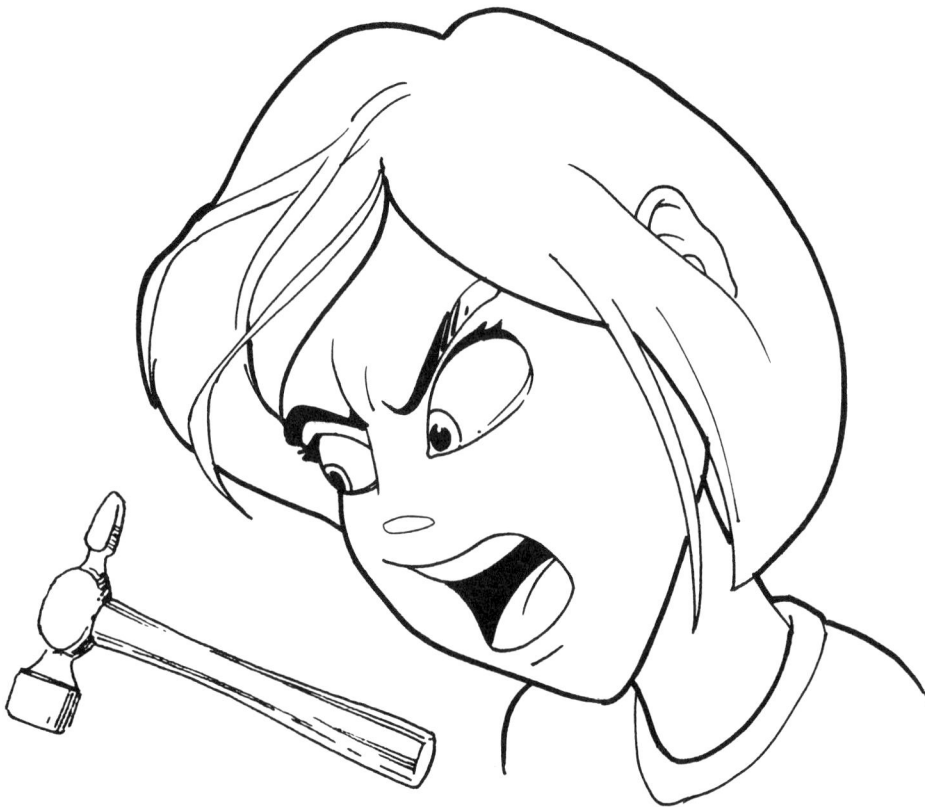

AVOID HARD ATTACKS

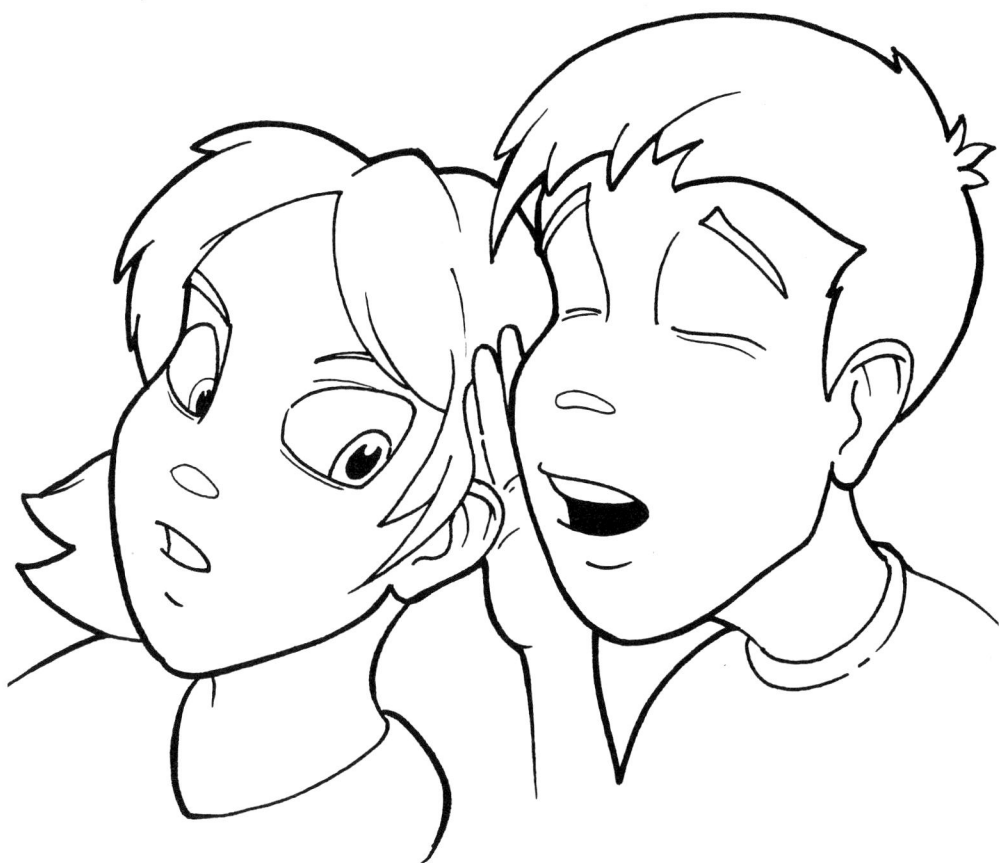

AVOID WHISPERING

APPENDIX 8 – BODY OUTLINE, VOICE BOX AND LUNGS

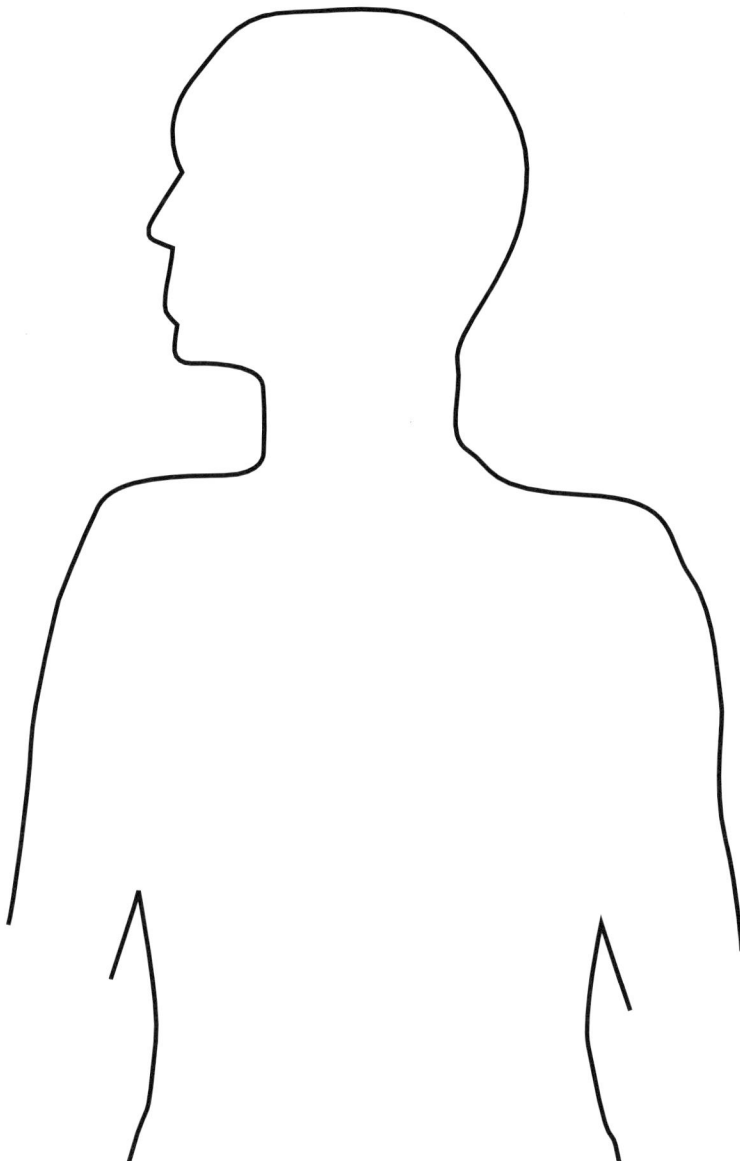

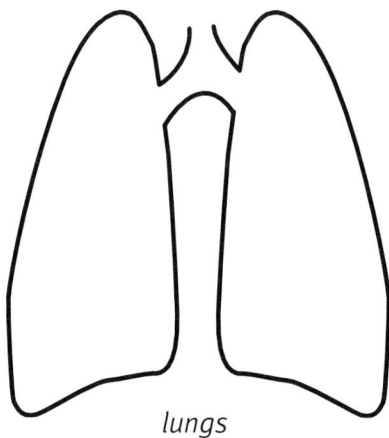

voice box

lungs

APPENDIX 9A – REFERRAL ACKNOWLEDGEMENT TO PARENT

SPEECH and LANGUAGE THERAPY SERVICE

Date _____

Dear Parent/Guardian of _____

A referral from _____ has been
received for a possible place in the Children's Voice Group.

An appointment for assessment will be sent to you within the next six weeks.

Yours sincerely

Speech & Language Therapist

APPENDIX 9B – REFERRAL ACKNOWLEDGEMENT TO REFERRER

SPEECH and LANGUAGE THERAPY SERVICE

Date _____

Dear _____

Thank you for referring _____

Hospital number _____

Date of birth _____

Address _____

_____

An appointment for assessment will be sent within the next six weeks.

Yours sincerely

Speech & Language Therapist

APPENDIX 9C – INITIAL APPOINTMENT LETTER

SPEECH and LANGUAGE THERAPY SERVICE

Date _____

Dear Parent/Guardian

An assessment appointment has been made for _____

on _____ at _____

Please return the slip below by _____ to confirm

attendance, otherwise the appointment will be given to another child.

Yours sincerely

Speech & Language Therapist

Please tick the appropriate box

Name of child _____

I will attend on _____ at _____ ☐

I am unable to attend, but would like another appointment. ☐

I no longer require an appointment. ☐

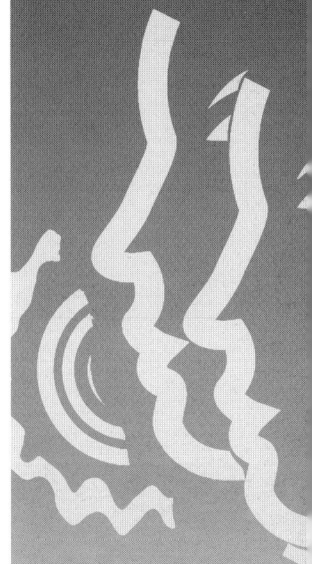
APPENDIX 9D – INITIAL ASSESSMENT REPORT

SPEECH and LANGUAGE THERAPY SERVICE

Date _____

INITIAL ASSESSMENT REPORT

Name _____ Hospital number _____

Date of birth _____

Address _____

GP _____

School _____

Referred by _____ Referral date _____

Comments

_____

_____

_____

Recommendations

_____

_____

_____

Speech & Language Therapist

Copies to _____

APPENDIX 9E – GROUP APPOINTMENT LETTER

SPEECH and LANGUAGE THERAPY SERVICE

Date _____

CHILDREN'S VOICE GROUP

To Parent / Guardian of _____

A place has been reserved in the Children's Voice Group, which will run on:

_____

_____

_____

_____

From _____ to _____

Please return the slip below by _____ to confirm attendance, otherwise the place will be offered to another child.

Yours sincerely

Speech & Language Therapist

Name _____

I will / will not * take up the place in the Children's Voice Group.

* *Delete as appropriate.*

APPENDIX 9F – LETTER TO SCHOOL

SPEECH and LANGUAGE THERAPY SERVICE

CHILDREN'S VOICE GROUP

Date _____

Dear Headteacher

Re _____

of _____

Date of birth _____

The above child attended for an assessment of their voice and has been given a programme to follow. Please find a copy enclosed.

It would be very helpful if this programme could be supported in school and a star chart completed.

He / she has been offered four appointments for therapy on:

_____ from _____ to _____

_____ from _____ to _____

_____ from _____ to _____

_____ from _____ to _____

Please contact the department if you have any queries.

Yours sincerely

Speech & Language Therapist

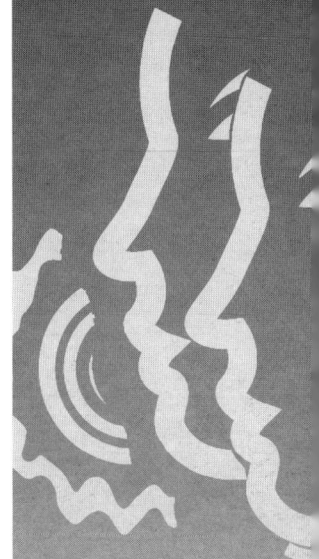

APPENDIX 9G – GROUP RECORD SHEET

PAEDIATRIC VOICE GROUP RECORD

Name: _____

Date _____
Date _____
Date _____
Date _____

Summary

9H
Working with
Children's Voice Disorders

SPEECH and LANGUAGE THERAPY SERVICE

Date _____

CHILDREN'S VOICE GROUP – THERAPY UPDATE

Name _____ Hospital number _____

Date of birth _____

Address _____

GP _____

School _____

Referred by _____ Referral date _____

Therapy summary

_____

_____

_____

Recommendations

_____

_____

_____

Speech & Language Therapist

Copies to _____

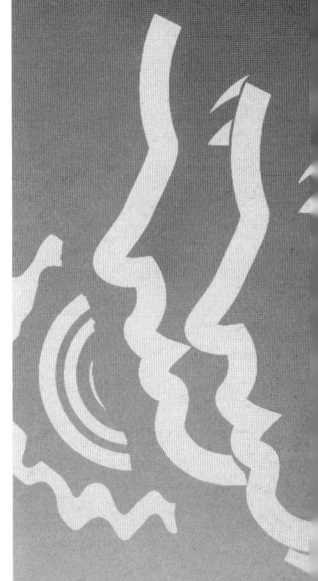

APPENDIX 9I – REVIEW APPOINTMENT LETTER

SPEECH and LANGUAGE THERAPY SERVICE

Date _____

CHILDREN'S VOICE GROUP

To Parent / Guardian of _____

A review appointment has been made on _____ at

_____

Please let me know if this is not convenient. If you do not attend, I shall assume that you feel _____ no longer requires Speech and Language Therapy.

Yours sincerely

Speech & Language Therapist

APPENDIX 9J – REVIEW REPORT

SPEECH and LANGUAGE THERAPY SERVICE

Date _____

CHILDREN'S VOICE GROUP – REVIEW REPORT

Name _____ Hospital number _____

Date of birth _____

Address _____

GP _____

School _____

Referred by _____ Referral date _____

Comments

_____

_____

_____

Recommendations

_____

_____

_____

Speech & Language Therapist

Copies to _____

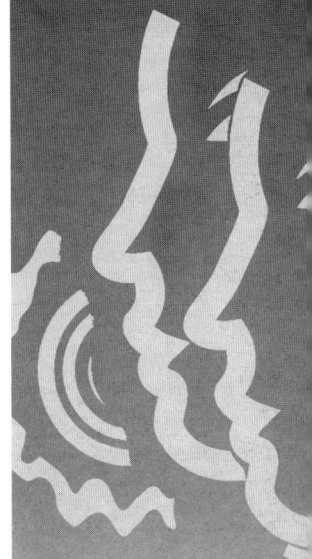

APPENDIX 9K – FAILURE TO ATTEND REVIEW LETTER

SPEECH and LANGUAGE THERAPY SERVICE

Date _____

Dear _____

Re _____

Address _____

Date of birth _____

Hospital number _____

Patient number _____

Following your referral of the above child for assessment of their voice, an appointment was sent for _____ at _____.

Unfortunately they did not attend or contact the clinic. A new appointment will not be sent unless they are re-referred in writing.

Yours sincerely

Speech & Language Therapist

Bibliography

Andrews M, 1986, *Voice Therapy for Children,* Singular Publishing, San Diego.

Andrews M, 1999, *The Manual of Voice Treatment: Pediatrics Through Geriatrics,* Singular Publishing, San Diego.

Andrews M, 2001, 'Paediatric and Adolescent Voice and Voice Disorders: Assessment, Management and Research', Seminar: Royal College of Surgeons, London.

Bagnell A, 1982, 'Panel Discussion', Lawrence VL (ed), *Transcripts of the 11th Symposium: Care of the Professional Voice,* The Voice Foundation, New York.

Boliek CA, Hixon TJ, Watson PJ & Morgan WJ, 1997, 'Vocalisation and Breathing During the Second and Third Years of Life', *Journal of Voice* 11(4), pp373–90.

Boone D, 1980, *The Boone Voice Program for Children*, CC Publications, Oregon.

Carding P, 2000, *Evaluating Voice Therapy,* Whurr Publishers, London.

ColorCards®, *Listening Skills (Indoor Sounds & Outdoor Sounds)*, Speechmark Publishing, Bicester.

ColorCards®, *Verbs series (Basic Verbs; Verbs & Verb Tenses)*, Speechmark Publishing, Bicester.

Colton RH & Casper JK, 1990, *Understanding Voice Problems*, Williams & Wilkins, Baltimore.

Cornut G & Troillet-Cornut A, 1995, 'Childhood dysphonia: clinical and therapeutic considerations', *Journal of British Voice Association* 4, pp70–76.

Cotes JE, 1979, *Lung Function,* 4th edn, Blackwell Scientific, Oxford.

Dahl, R, 2001, *Revolting Rhymes*, Puffin Books, London.

Deem JF & Miller L, 2000, *Manual of Voice Therapy,* Pro-ed Inc, Texas.

Enderby P, 1997, *Therapy Outcome Measures*, Singular Publishing, London.

Estill J, 1995, *Voicecraft: A User's Guide to Voice Quality*, Vol 2, Estill Voice Training Systems, Santa Rosa, California.

Green G, 1989, 'Pyscho-behavioural Characteristics of Children with Vocal Nodules: WPBIC Ratings', *Journal of Speech and Hearing Disorder* 54, pp306–12.

Greene MCL, 1980, *The Voice and its Disorders,* Pitman Medical, London.

Harris T, Harris S, Rubin JS & Howard DM, 2000, *The Voice Clinic Handbook,* Whurr Publishers, London.

Hirano M, 1981, *Clinical Examination of Voice,* Springer-Verlag, Vienna.

Hirano M, 1991, 'Phonosurgical Anatomy of the Larynx', in Nord C & Bless DM (eds), *Phonosurgery: Assessment of Voice Disorders,* Raven Press, New York.

Hirano M, Kurita S & Nakashima T, 1983, 'Growth, Development and Aging of Human Vocal Folds', Bless DM & Abbs JH (eds), *Vocal Fold Physiology,* College-Hill Press, San Diego.

Hunt J & Slater A, 1995, 'Children with Voice Disorders: The Benefits of a Group Approach', *RCSLT Bulletin* 520, pp12–13.

Hunt J & Slater A, 1996, 'Child Dysphonia – Harmony and Balance', *Speech and Language Therapy in Practice* 5(4), pp21–3.

Hunt J & Slater A, 1999, 'From to Start to Outcome and Beyond', *Speech and Language Therapy in Practice*, Autumn, pp4–6.

Jones SEM, Hunt J & Pickles J, nd, 'Is Ethnicity a Cause of Paediatric Dysphonia?', unpublished manuscript. Available from Luton and Dunstable Hospital Voice Clinic, Bedfordshire.

Kahane JC & Kahn AR, 1984, 'Weight Measurements of Infant and Adult Intrinsic Laryngeal Muscles', *Folia Phoniatrica* 36, p129.

Kahane JC & Mayo R, 1989, 'The Need for Aggressive Pursuit on Healthy Childhood Voices', *Language, Speech and Hearing Services in Schools* 20, pp102–7.

Kay NJ, 1982, 'Vocal Nodules in Children – Aetiology and Management', *Journal of Laryngology and Otology* 96(8), pp731–6.

Laver J, Wirz S & MacKenzie J, 1982, 'Vocal Profile Analysis Protocol', *Vocal Profiles of Speech Disorders Research Project,* University of Edinburgh Press, Edinburgh.

MacLarnon AM & Hewitt GP, 1999, 'The Evolution of Human Speech: The Role of Enhanced Breathing Control', *The American Journal of Physical Anthropology* 109(3), pp341–63.

Maddern BR, Thomas MD, Campbell F & Sylvan Stool, 1991, 'Paediatric voice disorders' *Otolaryngologic Clinics of North America* 24(5).

Martin S & Lockhart M, 2000, *Working with Voice Disorders,* Speechmark Publishing, Bicester.

Martin S & Darnley L, 1992, *The Voice Sourcebook,* Speechmark Publishing, Bicester.

Mathieson L, 2001, 'Voice Mutation, Infancy to Senescence', in Greene M and Mathieson L (eds) *The Voice and its Disorders,* 6th edn, Whurr Publishers, London.

McCrory E, 2001, 'Treating Vocal Nodules: Are We Measuring Up?', *RCSLT Bulletin,* 585 (January), pp10–11.

Miller S & Madison C, 1984, 'Public School Voice Clinics, Part 2: Diagnosis and Recommendations – a 10 year review', *American Speech Language and Hearing Association, Language, Speech and Hearing Services in Schools* 15(January) pp58–63.

Milligan, S, 1973, *Silly Verse for Kids*, Puffin Books, London.

Moran MJ & Pentz AL, 1987, 'Otolaryngologists' opinions of voice therapy for vocal nodules in children', *American Speech Language and Hearing Association, Language, Speech, and Hearing Services in Schools* 18, pp17–18.

Mori K, 1999, 'Vocal Fold Nodules in Children: Preferable Therapy', *International Journal of Pediatric Otorhinolaryngol* 49(Supplement 1), ppS303–6.

Niedziesla G, Wroczek-Glijer E & Toman D, 2000, 'Voice Disorders in Children with Gastroesophageal Reflux Disease', *Otolarygol Pol* 54(1), pp67–8.

Pannbacker M, 1998, 'Voice Treatment Techniques: A Review and Recommendations for Outcome Studies', *American Journal of Speech-Language Pathology* 7(3), pp49–64.

Pannbacker M, 1999, 'Treatment of Vocal Nodules: Options and Outcomes', *American Journal of Speech-Language Pathology* 8, pp209–17.

Ramig LO & Verdolini KM, 1998, 'Treatment Efficacy: Voice Disorders', *Journal of Speech, Language, and Hearing Research* 41, ppS101–16.

Rattenbury H, 2001, 'Can SLTs Afford Not to be Doing their Own Fibreoptic Nasendoscopy?', paper delivered at Newcastle Voice Conference, Freeman Hospital, Newcastle.

Sander EK, 1989, 'Arguments Against the Aggressive Pursuit of Voice Therapy for Children', *Language, Speech, and Hearing Services in Schools* 20(1), pp94–101.

Sarfati J & Auday T, 1996, 'Course of benign dysphonia in children', *Rev. Laryngol. Otol. Rhinol. (Bord)* 117(4), pp327–9.

Schalen L & Rydell R, 1995, 'Dysphonia in Children: Not Necessarily Due to Voice Abuse', *Journal of British Voice Association* 4, pp44–56.

Sheppard WC & Lane HI, 1968, 'Development of Prosodic Features of Infant Vocalising', *Journal of Speech and Hearing Research* 11, p94.

Stone RE, 1982, 'Management of Childhood Dysphonias of Organic Bases', Filter MD (ed), *Phonatory Voice Disorders in Children,* Charles C Thomas, Springfield, Illinois.

Thyme-Frøkjær K & Frøkjær-Jensen B, 2001, *The Accent Method*, Speechmark Publishing, Bicester.

Verdolini K, Ramig L & Jacobson B, 1997, 'Outcome Measurements in Voice Disorders', in Frattali CM (ed), *Measuring Outcomes in Speech-Language Pathology*, Thieme, New York.

Von Leden H, 1985, 'Vocal nodules in children', *Ear, Nose, and Throat Journal* 64, pp473–80.

Ward S & Birkett D, 1992, ' The predictive validity and accuracy of a screening test for language delay and auditory perceptual disorder', *European Journal of Disorders of Communication* 27, pp55–72.

West JB, 1979, *Respiratory Physiology*, 2nd edn, Williams & Wilkins, Baltimore.

White P, 1995, 'Some Acoustic Measurements of Children's Voiced and Whispered Vowels', *Journal of the British Voice Association* 4, pp1–15.

Wilson DK, 1987, *Voice Problems of Children*, 3rd edn, Williams & Wilkins, Baltimore.

World Health Organisation, 1980, *International Classification of Impairments, Disabilities, Handicaps: A manual for Classification Relating to the Consequences of Disease*, WHO, Geneva.

Working with . . . the Complete Series

In dealing with day-to-day management of clients, the Speechmark Working with . . . series has established an enviable reputation as the essential resource for every speech and language professional. The following titles are available:

Working with
Adults with a Learning Disability
Alex Kelly

This comprehensive and practical resource covers all aspects of working with adults with a learning disability. Topics covered include: assessment of clients and their environment; profound and multiple disability; challenging behaviour; augmentative and alternative communication; social skills and dysphagia. In addition the author addresses staff training, group therapy, accessing the criminal justice system and working within a multidisciplinary team. A revised version of the author's popular *Personal Communication Plan* is included.

Working with
Children's Language
Jackie Cooke & Diana Williams

Containing a wealth of ideas and a wide range of activities, the practical approach to language teaching has helped establish this book as a leading manual in its field. Games, activities and ideas suitable for developing specific language skills make this handbook a valuable resource for everyone working with children.

Working with
Children's Phonology
Gwen Lancaster & Lesley Pope

Successfully bridging the gap between theory and practice, this book provides a wealth of creative ideas for lively and entertaining activities for therapy. This thoroughly practical manual also examines recent advances in the analysis and description of phonological disorders and describes their management within the clinic.

Working with
Children's Voice Disorders
Jenny Hunt & Alyson Slater

A practical resource book intended for speech & language therapists and students who have little

previous experience of working with children with dysphonia, enabling therapists to work confidently and to gain the necessary skills to manage this client group within their generic caseload.

Contains ideas for setting up treatment groups, case studies and suggestions on how to evaluate therapy and measure outcomes.

Working with
Dysarthrics
Sandra Robertson & Fay Thomson

This is a unique source of ideas for individual and group speech therapy with patients who have dysarthria as a result of acquired neurological damage.

Current theory on the problems of dysarthria and assessment procedures as well as the principles, goals and efficacy of treatment are discussed. These are linked with practical activities and large print exercises to improve all aspects of motor speech.

Working with
Dysfluent Children
Trudy Stewart & Jackie Turnbull

This essential manual analyses dysfluency in children and provides the reader with practical ways of handling these difficulties in collaboration with the child, parents and carers.

Complete with case studies, key summaries, notes on teaching the easy onset technique, lists of therapy resources and a comprehensive index, this text will be an essential reference for all those involved in working with dysfluent children.

Working with
Oral Cancer
Julia Appleton & Jane Machin

This addition to the series presents clinicians with a practical working knowledge of swallowing and speech disorders arising as a result of surgery for carcinoma of the oral cavity.

With very little written matter presently available on this specialist subject area, this title will be invaluable to therapists and students who wish to develop new skills or would like to build on existing knowledge.

Working with
Pragmatics
Lucie Andersen-Wood & Benita Rae Smith

Covering the principles and practice of pragmatics and firmly grounded in theory, this title contains practical teaching activities to help develop communication skills. Assessment and diagnostic measures are also provided. The appendices contain a useful literature review and a list of the characteristics of pragmatic dysfunction. There are also photocopiable materials including a client-centred assessment form and child and client information sheets. A comprehensive bibliography and index complete this excellent resource. A ground-breaking title written by speech & language therapists who have also worked together as senior lecturers on this topic.

Working with
Voice Disorders
Stephanie Martin & Myra Lockhart

This new title provides an essential resource for clinicians of varying levels of experience from student to specialist. It follows the client's journey along the health continuum from disorder back to health, providing practical insights and direction in all aspects of patient management. The authors provide a sound theoretical framework to this specialism and offer a rich variety of photocopiable, practical resource material.

The multi-dimensional structure of the book allows the clinician to examine specific aspects of patient management, as well as issues of clinical effectiveness, clinical governance and service management. The clinician-friendly, patient-centred approach makes this an essential resource.

These are just a few of the many therapy resources available from Speechmark.

Related Resources

Children's Phonology Sourcebook by Lesley Flynn & Gwen Lancaster;
Dysarthria Sourcebook by Sandra Robertson, Barbara Tanner & Fay Young;
Dysfluency Resource Book by Jackie Turnbull & Trudy Stewart;
The Voice Sourcebook by Stephanie Martin & Lyn Darnley.

Speechmark